Lecture Notes in Computer Science 10038

Commenced Publication in 1973
Founding and Former Series Editors:
Gerhard Goos, Juris Hartmanis, and Jan van Leeuwen

Editorial Board

David Hutchison
Lancaster University, Lancaster, UK
Takeo Kanade
Carnegie Mellon University, Pittsburgh, PA, USA
Josef Kittler
University of Surrey, Guildford, UK
Jon M. Kleinberg
Cornell University, Ithaca, NY, USA
Friedemann Mattern
ETH Zurich, Zurich, Switzerland
John C. Mitchell
Stanford University, Stanford, CA, USA
Moni Naor
Weizmann Institute of Science, Rehovot, Israel
C. Pandu Rangan
Indian Institute of Technology, Madras, India
Bernhard Steffen
TU Dortmund University, Dortmund, Germany
Demetri Terzopoulos
University of California, Los Angeles, CA, USA
Doug Tygar
University of California, Berkeley, CA, USA
Gerhard Weikum
Max Planck Institute for Informatics, Saarbrücken, Germany

More information about this series at http://www.springer.com/series/7409

Xiaoxia Yin · James Geller
Ye Li · Rui Zhou
Hua Wang · Yanchun Zhang (Eds.)

Health Information Science

5th International Conference, HIS 2016
Shanghai, China, November 5–7, 2016
Proceedings

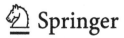 Springer

Editors

Xiaoxia Yin
Centre for Applied Informatics
Victoria University
Melbourne
Australia

Rui Zhou
Centre for Applied Informatics
Victoria University
Melbourne
Australia

James Geller
Computer Science
New Jersey Institute of Technology
Newark, NJ
USA

Hua Wang
Centre for Applied Informatics
Victoria University
Melbourne
Australia

Ye Li
Shenzhen Institute of Advanced Technology
Chinese Academy of Sciences
Shenzhen
China

Yanchun Zhang
Centre for Applied Informatics
Victoria University
Melbourne
Australia

ISSN 0302-9743   ISSN 1611-3349   (electronic)
Lecture Notes in Computer Science
ISBN 978-3-319-48334-4   ISBN 978-3-319-48335-1   (eBook)
DOI 10.1007/978-3-319-48335-1

Library of Congress Control Number: 2016954942

LNCS Sublibrary: SL3 – Information Systems and Applications, incl. Internet/Web, and HCI

This Springer imprint is published by Springer Nature
The registered company is Springer International Publishing AG
The registered company address is: Gewerbestrasse 11, 6330 Cham, Switzerland

Preface

The International Conference Series on Health Information Science (HIS) provides a forum for disseminating and exchanging multidisciplinary research results in computer science/information technology and health science and services. It covers all aspects of health information sciences and systems that support health information management and health service delivery.

The 5th International Conference on Health Information Science (HIS 2016) was held in Shanghai, China, during November 5–7, 2016. Founded in April 2012 as the International Conference on Health Information Science and Their Applications, the conference continues to grow to include an ever broader scope of activities. The main goal of these events is to provide international scientific forums for researchers to exchange new ideas in a number of fields that interact in-depth through discussions with their peers from around the world. The scope of the conference includes: (1) medical/health/biomedicine information resources, such as patient medical records, devices and equipment, software and tools to capture, store, retrieve, process, analyze, and optimize the use of information in the health domain, (2) data management, data mining, and knowledge discovery, all of which play a key role in decision-making, management of public health, examination of standards, privacy, and security issues, (3) computer visualization and artificial intelligence for computer-aided diagnosis, and (4) development of new architectures and applications for health information systems.

The conference solicited and gathered technical research submissions related to all aspects of the conference scope. All the submitted papers in the proceeding were peer reviewed by at least three international experts drawn from the Program Committee. After the rigorous peer-review process, a total of 13 full papers and nine short papers among 44 submissions were selected on the basis of originality, significance, and clarity and were accepted for publication in the proceedings. The authors were from seven countries, including Australia, China, France, The Netherlands, Thailand, the UK, and USA. Some authors were invited to submit extended versions of their papers to a special issue of the *Health Information Science and System* journal, published by BioMed Central (Springer) and the *World Wide Web* journal.

The high quality of the program — guaranteed by the presence of an unparalleled number of internationally recognized top experts — can be assessed when reading the contents of the proceeding. The conference was therefore a unique event, where attendees were able to appreciate the latest results in their field of expertise and to acquire additional knowledge in other fields. The program was structured to favor interactions among attendees coming from many different horizons, scientifically and geographically, from academia and from industry.

We would like to sincerely thank our keynote and invited speakers:

- Professor Ling Liu, Distributed Data Intensive Systems Lab, School of Computer Science, Georgia Institute of Technology, USA

- Professor Lei Liu, Institution of Biomedical Research, Fudan University; Deputy director of Biological Information Technology Research Center, Shanghai, China
- Professor Uwe Aickelin, Faculty of Science, University of Nottingham, UK
- Professor Ramamohanarao (Rao) Kotagiri, Department of Computing and Information Systems, The University of Melbourne, Australia
- Professor Fengfeng Zhou, College of Computer Science and Technology, Jilin University, China
- Associate Professor Hongbo Ni, School of Computer Science, Northwestern Polytechnical University, China

Our thanks also go to the host organization, Fudan University, China, and the support of the National Natural Science Foundation of China (No. 61332013) for funding. Finally, we acknowledge all those who contributed to the success of HIS 2016 but whose names are not listed here.

November 2016   Xiaoxia Yin
                                                                James Geller
                                                                      Ye Li
                                                                  Rui Zhou
                                                                 Hua Wang
                                                            Yanchun Zhang

Organization

General Co-chairs

Lei Liu   Fudan University, China
Uwe Aickelin   The University of Nottingham, UK
Yanchun Zhang   Victoria University, Australia and Fudan University,
                            China

Program Co-chairs

Xiaoxia Yin   Victoria University, Australia
James Geller   New Jersey Institute of Technology, USA
Ye Li   Shenzhen Institutes of Advanced Technology,
                            Chinese Academy of Sciences, China

Conference Organization Chair

Hua Wang   Victoria University, Australia

Industry Program Chair

Chaoyi Pang   Zhejiang University, China

Workshop Chair

Haolan Zhang   Zhejiang University, China

Publication and Website Chair

Rui Zhou   Victoria University, Australia

Publicity Chair

Juanying Xie   Shaanxi Normal University, China

Local Arrangements Chair

Shanfeng Zhu   Fudan University, China

Finance Co-chairs

Lanying Zhang   Fudan University, China
Irena Dzuteska   Victoria University, Australia

Program Committee

Mathias Baumert   The University of Adelaide, Australia
Jiang Bian   University of Florida, USA
Olivier Bodenreider   U.S. National Library of Medicine, USA
David Buckeridge   McGill University, Canada
Ilvio Bruder   Universität Rostock, Germany
Klemens Böhm   Karlsruhe Institute of Technology, Germany
Jinhai Cai   University of South Australia, Australia
Yunpeng Cai   Shenzhen Institutes of Advanced Technology,
                           Chinese Academy of Sciences, China
Jeffrey Chan   The University of Melbourne, Australia
Fei Chen   South University of Science and Technology of China,
                           China
Song Chen   University of Maryland, Baltimore County, USA
Wei Chen   Fudan University, China
You Chen   Vanderbilt University, USA
Soon Ae Chun   The City University of New York, USA
Jim Cimino   National Institutes of Health, USA
Carlo Combi   University of Verona, Italy
Licong Cui   Case Western Reserve University, USA
Peng Dai   University of Toronto, Canada
Xuan-Hong Dang   University of California at Santa Barbara, USA
Hongli Dong   Northeast Petroleum University, China
Ling Feng   Tsinghua University, China
Kin Wah Fung   National Library of Medicine, USA
Sillas Hadjiloucas   University of Reading, UK
Zhe He   Florida State University, USA
Zhisheng Huang   Vrije Universiteit Amsterdam, The Netherlands
Du Huynh   The University of Western Australia, Australia
Guoqian Jiang   Mayo Clinic College of Medicine, USA
Xia Jing   Ohio University, USA
Jiming Liu   Hong Kong Baptist University, Hong Kong,
                           SAR China
Gang Luo   University of Utah, USA
Zhiyuan Luo   Royal Holloway, University of London, UK
Nigel Martin   Birkbeck, University of London, UK
Fernando Martin-Sanchez Weill Cornell Medicine, USA
Sally Mcclean   Ulster University, UK
Bridget Mcinnes   Virginia Commonwealth University, USA
Fleur Mougin   ERIAS, ISPED, U897, France

Contents

Real-Time Patient Table Removal in CT Images

Luming Chen[1,2], Shibin Wu[1,3(✉)], Zhicheng Zhang[1,3], Shaode Yu[1,3],
Yaoqin Xie[1], and Hefang Zhang[2]

[1] Shenzhen Institutes of Advanced Technology,
Chinese Academy of Sciences, Shenzhen 518055, China
{lm.chen,sb.wu,zc.zhang,sd.yu,yq.xie}@siat.ac.cn
[2] College of Electrical and Information Engineering,
Xi'An Technological University, Xi'an 710021, China
dzxzhf@163.com
[3] Shenzhen College of Advanced Technology,
University of Chinese Academy of Sciences, Shenzhen 518055, China
http://www.siat.ac.cn/

Abstract. As a routine tool for screening and examination, CT plays
an important role in disease detection and diagnosis. Real-time table
removal in CT images becomes a fundamental task to improve readability, interpretation and treatment planning. Meanwhile, it makes data
management simple and benefits information sharing and communication in picture archiving and communication system. In this paper, we
proposed an automated framework which utilized parallel programming
to address this problem. Eight full-body CT images were collected and
analyzed. Experimental results have shown that with parallel programming, the proposed framework can accelerate the patient table removal
task up to three times faster when it was running on a personal computer with four-core central processing unit. Moreover, the segmentation
accuracy reaches 99 % of Dice coefficient. The idea behind this approach
refreshes many algorithms for real-time medical image processing without extra hardware spending.

Keywords: Real-time · Parallel programming · Image segmentation ·
Health information science

1 Introduction

In spite of the use of MRI in clinical imaging, CT becomes more common in
routine screening and examination [1–4]. The usage of CT scanning has increased
impressively over the last two decades [5]. It visualizes body structures vividly,
such as head, lung and cardiac, and produce huge amounts of data which imposes
difficulties on data management, information sharing and communication.

In clinical applications, a fundamental task is patient table removal. It aims
to localize and remove the table from CT images [6]. Subsequently, it enhances

© Springer International Publishing AG 2016
X. Yin et al. (Eds.): HIS 2016, LNCS 10038, pp. 1–8, 2016.
DOI: 10.1007/978-3-319-48335-1_1

tissue visualization [7], improves the accuracy in information fusion [8–12]. Meanwhile, it makes data management simple and further benefits information sharing and communication [13,14]. However, literatures on patient table removal is scarce, mainly because vendors have implemented these algorithms in the software platform and give no interface to users.

Methods for table removal can be grouped into manual, semi-automatic and automatic. Manual delineation is time consuming, laborious and biased. Semi-automatic techniques allow users incorporating prior knowledge in the segmentation procedure and lessens time cost [15,16]. But with respect to a full-body CT volume with hundreds of slices, it is again laborious and boring. Therefore, automated methods are more appealing and promising. Automated CT table removal is challenging, because different vendors supply different CT scanning tables with their unique characteristics. Based on the observation that the table top forms a straight line in sagittal planes while the table cross-section is almost invariant axially, Zhu *et al.* [6] developed an automated method utilizing Hough transformation [17].

In this paper, we proposed an automated framework. It utilized parallel programming and proper algorithm deployment for real-time table removal. The remainder of this paper is organized as follows. Section 2 describes the framework for patient table removal, including algorithm implementation and parallel programming. Sections 3 and 4 presents experimental results from segmentation accuracy and acceleration factor. This study is summarized in Sect. 4.

2   Methods and Materials

2.1   Proposed Framework

The proposed framework mainly involves image binarization and morphological operation as shown in Fig. 1. First, one image slice as the input is binaried with Otsu thresholding method [18]. Then the foreground, the body and the table are extracted while holes in the foreground region are filled. After that, morphological opening operation is used to remove the table structure and isolate the body part in binary foreground region. Finally, the table is removed and the algorithm outcome is a mask that contains only body regions.

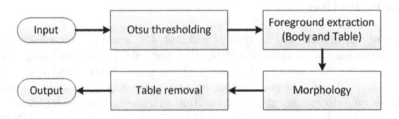

Fig. 1. Semantic description of the proposed framework. It employs simple algorithms (Otsu thresholding and morphological operation).

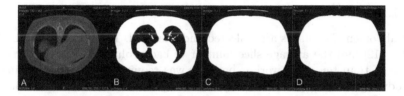

Fig. 2. An example for the proposed framework. (A) is the input, (B) is after Otsu thresholding, (C) is after morphological operation and (D) is the mask for the outcome.

Figure 2 shows a representative example to describe the proposed framework. A slice as the input is shown in (A) and then binarized with Otsu method (B). Then morphological operation is borrowed for filling holes and completes the body regions (C). In the end, the table is removed (D).

2.2 Parallel Programming

With the development of hardware and software, algorithm acceleration is widely used. It can be realized with parallel programming either on graphic processing unit (GPU) or on multi-core CPU [19,20]. However, in practice, GPU-based acceleration is difficult for algorithm deployment and leads to extra spending. On the contrary, parallel programming based on multi-core CPU is more promising because of its technical maturity and ease of use. In particular, personal computers with multi-core CPU are easy accessible. Motivated by [21], we utilized multi-core CPU based parallel programming for real-time CT table removal.

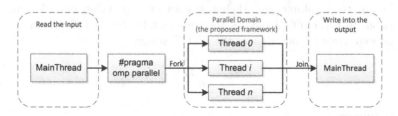

Fig. 3. The parallel programming strategy. After reading in the CT volume, slices are processed with multi-threads running on different CPU so that time is lessened. (Color figure online)

The scheme of parallel programming can be divided into three parts as shown in Fig. 3. The most important part is in the parallel domain (the red section). After reading in the volume image, the parallel-thread number is determined by the CPU processers and the proposed framework shown in Fig. 1 is running at each thread. Finally, all processed image slices are written and saved. In the scheme, the memory is shared in computation.

2.3   Experiment Design

Eight abdomen CT images are collected and analyzed. The in-plane matrix size is [512, 512] and the average slice number to each volume is 120. A physician with more than ten years work experience was required to manually delineate the body region slice by slice and built a solid ground truth for validation.

2.4   Performance Criteria

As CT table removal is equal to whole-body segmentation, the performance is quantified from body segmentation. First, $DICE$ coefficient is used to evaluate volume overlaps between the segmentation result (S) and the ground truth (G). Its value is in [0, 1] and higher values indicate better segmentation. $DICE$ coefficient is defined in Eq. 1.

$$DICE = 2\frac{|G \cap S|}{|G| + |S|}. \tag{1}$$

Meanwhile, false positive (FP) and false negative (FN) errors are computed, respectively in Eqs. 2 and 3. Note that in Eqs. 1 to 3, $|\cdot|$ indicates the volume computed as the number of voxels.

$$FP = \frac{|S| - |G \cap S|}{|G|}, \tag{2}$$

$$FN = \frac{|G| - |G \cap S|}{|G|}. \tag{3}$$

In addition, the real-time ability is concerned. It first records a total time consumption to a volume and then takes an average value per slice for fair comparison. In Eq. 4, TC_i indicates the time cost to the ith CT volume and tc_i is the average time for one slice in the ith CT volume.

$$tc_i = \frac{1}{n}TC_i \tag{4}$$

2.5   Software

All codes are implemented on VS2010 (https://www.visualstudio.com/) and running on a workstation with 4 Intel (R) Cores (TM) of 3.70 GHz and 8 GB DDR RAM. Involved third-party softwares are OpenMP (http://openmp.org/wp/), OpenCV (http://opencv.org/) and ITK (http://www.itk.org/).

3   Results and Discussion

3.1   Segmentation Accuracy

Table removal accuracy is verified from $DICE$, FP and FN shown in Fig. 4. It is observed that the $DICE$ value is very close to 1 (Mean value, 99.14 %).

That means, the proposed framework is very effective and precise. Moreover, FP indicates that very less voxels outside the patient body is wrongly isolated into the body region (Mean value, 0.04 %). In addition, only about 1.63 % of voxels in the body region is omitted. Hence, the proposed framework can remove patient table accurately and robustly.

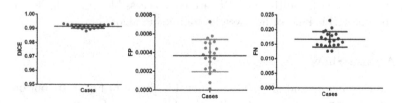

Fig. 4. Table removal accuracy. The average value of $DICE$, FP and FN is 99.14 %, 0.04 % and 1.63 %, respectively. It shows the proposed scheme is feasible and effective.

The precision of patient table removal or body segmentation is important. It relates to image registration, disease detection, pattern interpretation and clinical diagnosis. Our framework is simple and produces accurate segmentation results. On one side, it isolates the regions of human body from the background and emphasizes physicians' attention on organs but not the table. On the other side, after patient table removal, the data saves about 1/4 to 1/3 disk space and benefits data archiving, sharing and communication (PACS) in health information system (HIS).

3.2   Real-Time Ability

The real-time ability of the proposed framework is concerned. It is compared to manual segmentation and the framework without parallel programming. Average time consumption to each slice is shown in Table 1. Please note that "Acc factor" stands for accelerated factor.

Table 1. Average time cost to each slice. When taken the time cost of proposed parallel framework as the baseline (=1.0), the acceleration factor is 429 and 2.72 for the manual and the proposed framework without parallel programming, respectively.

	Manual	No parallel	Parallel
Time cost	124.51	0.79	0.29
Acc factor	429.34	2.72	1.0

The real-time ability is severely underestimated in clinic. Some algorithms prolong the waiting time and may upset patients. Based on existing hardware and without extra spending, the proposed framework will dramatically accelerate the image segmentation procedure with more CPU cores and fine algorithm implementation. Compared to manual delineation, it speeds up to 430 times faster; while compared to serial processing, it accelerates the procedure up to 2.7 times on a four-core CPU. With a professional computer, the acceleration factor ("Acc factor") could be more impressive. GPU-based acceleration is also desirable. However, it needs additional hardware and more complex algorithm deployment. That means, time and money should be supplemented. While nowadays, computers with multi-core CPU are easy accessible. As such, it is meaningful to deploy this kind of lightweight computing algorithm.

3.3 A Case Show

A clinical case before and after table removal is shown in Fig. 5. It contains 163 slices with in-plane resolution of [512, 512]. The original CT image is shown in the top row and the bottom shows the image after the table is removed.

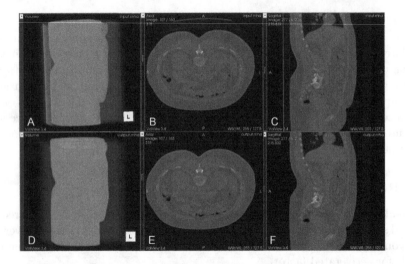

Fig. 5. A clinical case before and after patient table removal. The top row shows the original CT image and the bottom is visualized after the table is removed.

In Fig. 5, (A, D) shows rendered volume surface, and the impact of the patient table is clearly seen by comparison. (B) is axial plane where the table is similar to two arc in the top region of the image and (C) shows the sagittal plane in which the top of the table forms two vertical lines paralleling to each other.

Since this collection is related to abdomen CT imaging, two limitations of the proposed algorithm may be mentioned. First of all, to a whole-body CT image, the algorithm might fail because of the head position and artifacts around as indicated in [6]. Secondly, the algorithm is simple and only validated on eight abdomen images. Thus, for general applications, some parameters or operations should be tuned.

4   Conclusion

An automatic framework for real-time table removal in CT images is proposed. It utilizes lightweight computing algorithms deployed with parallel programming. Eight abdomen CT images have verified its accuracy and real-time ability. This framework makes use of existing hardware and software without extra spending and benefits data storage, sharing and communication in health information system.

Acknowledgment. This work is supported by grants from National Natural Science Foundation of China (Grant No. 81501463), Guangdong Innovative Research Team Program (Grant No. 2011S013), National 863 Programs of China (Grant No. 2015AA043203), Shenzhen Fundamental Research Program (Grant Nos. JCYJ20140417113430726, JCYJ20140417113430665 and JCYJ201500731154850923) and Beijing Center for Mathematics and Information Interdisciplinary Sciences.

References

1. Mettler, Jr. F.A., Wiest, P.W., Locken, J.A., et al.: CT scanning: patterns of use and dose. J. Radiol. Protect. **20**(4), 353–359 (2000)
2. Li, T., Xing, L.: Optimizing 4D cone-beam CT acquisition protocol for external beam radiotherapy. Intl. J. Radiat. Oncol. Biol. Phys. **67**(4), 1211–1219 (2007)
3. Paquin, D., Levy, D., Xing, L.: Multiscale registration of planning CT and daily cone beam CT images for adaptive radiation therapy. Medical Phys. **36**(1), 4–11 (2009)
4. Xing, L., Wessels, B., Hendee, W.R.: The value of PET/CT is being over-sold as a clinical tool in radiation oncology. Medical Phys. **32**(6), 1457–1459 (2005)
5. Smith-Bindman, R., Lipson, J., Marcus, R., et al.: Radiation dose associated with common computed tomography examinations and the associated lifetime attributable risk of cancer. Arch. Internal Med. **169**(22), 2078–2086 (2009)
6. Zhu, Y.M., Cochoff, S.M., Sukalac, R.: Automatic patient table removal in CT images. J. Digital Imag. **169**(22), **25**(4), 480–485 (2012)
7. Kim, J., Hu, Y., Eberl, S., et al.: A fully automatic bed/linen segmentation for fused PET/CT MIP rendering. Soc. Nuclear Med. Ann. Meet. Abs. **49**(Supplement 1), 387 (2008)
8. Chao, M., Xie, Y., Xing, L.: Auto-propagation of contours for adaptive prostate radiation therapy. Phys. Med. Biol. **53**(17), 4533 (2008)
9. Xie, Y., Chao, M., Lee, P., et al.: Feature-based rectal contour propagation from planning CT to cone beam CT. Med. Phys. **35**(10), 4450–4459 (2008)
10. Schreibmann, E., Chen, G.T.Y., Xing, L.: Image interpolation in 4D CT using a BSpline deformable registration model. Intl. J. Radiat. Oncol. Biol. Phys. **64**(5), 1537–1550 (2006)
11. Mihaylov, I.B., Corry, P., Yan, Y., et al.: Modeling of carbon fiber couch attenuation properties with a commercial treatment planning system. Med. Phys. **35**(11), 4982–4988 (2008)
12. Zhang, R., Zhou, W., et al.: Nonrigid registration of lung CT images based on tissue features. Comput. Math. Methods Med. **2013**, 7 (2013)
13. Ammenwerth, E., Graber, S., Herrmann, G., et al.: Evaluation of health information systems - problems and challenges. Intl. J. Med. Inf. **71**(2), 125–135 (2003)

14. Haux, R.: Health information systems Cpast, present, future. Intl. J. Med. Inf. **75**(3), 268–281 (2006)
15. Zhou, W., Xie, Y.: Interactive contour delineation and refinement in treatment planning of image-guided radiation therapy. J. Appl. Clin. Med. Phys. **15**(1), 4499 (2014)
16. Zhou, W., Xie, Y.: Interactive medical image segmentation using snake and multiscale curve editing. Comput. Math. Methods Med. **2013**, 1–22 (2013)
17. Duda, R.O., Hart, P.E.: Use of the Hough transformation to detect lines and curves in pictures. Commun. ACM **15**(1), 11–15 (1972)
18. Otsu, N.: A threshold selection method from gray-level histograms. Automatica **11**(285–296), 23–27 (1975)
19. Du, P., Weber, R., et al.: From CUDA to OpenCL: Towards a performance-portable solution for multi-platform GPU programming. Parallel Comput. **38**(8), 391–407 (2012)
20. Brodtkorb, A.R., Hagen, T.R., et al.: Graphics processing unit (GPU) programming strategies and trends in GPU computing. J. Parallel Distrib. Comput. **73**(1), 4–13 (2013)
21. Wang, G., Zuluaga, M.A., Pratt, R., Aertsen, M., David, A.L., Deprest, J., Vercauteren, T., Ourselin, S.: Slic-seg: slice-by-slice segmentation propagation of the placenta in fetal MRI using one-plane scribbles and online learning. In: Navab, N., Hornegger, J., Wells, W.M., Frangi, A.F. (eds.) MICCAI 2015. LNCS, vol. 9351, pp. 29–37. Springer, Heidelberg (2015). doi:10.1007/978-3-319-24574-4_4

A Distributed Decision Support Architecture for the Diagnosis and Treatment of Breast Cancer

Liang Xiao[1(✉)] and John Fox[2]

[1] Hubei University of Technology, Wuhan, Hubei, China
lx@mail.hbut.edu.cn
[2] University of Oxford, Oxford, UK
john.fox@eng.ox.ac.uk

Abstract. Clinical decision support for the diagnosis and treatment of breast cancer needs to be provided for a multidisciplinary team to improve the care. The execution of clinical knowledge in an appropriate representation to support decisions, however, is typically centrally orchestrated and inconsistent with the nature and environment that specialists work together. The use of guideline language of PRO*forma* for breast cancer has been examined with the issues raised, and an agent-oriented distributed decision support architecture is put forward. The key components of this architecture include a goal-decomposition structure (shaping the architecture), agent planning rules (individual decision-making), and agent argumentation rules (reasoning among decision options). The shift from a centralised decision support solution to a distributed one is illustrated using the breast cancer scenario and this generic approach will be applied to a wider range of clinical problems in future.

Keywords: Agent · Breast cancer · Distributed clinical decision support · Goal · Rule

1 Introduction and Motivation

Breast cancer remains an important cause of morbidity and mortality around the world. One woman in 9 will develop breast cancer at some time during her lifetime, and breast cancer causes around 13,000 deaths per annum in the UK alone [1]. In improving outcomes in breast cancer, the very first key recommendation given by the Department of Health and the National Institute for Clinical Excellence is that, women should be treated by a multidisciplinary team of healthcare professionals having all the necessary skills [2]. This means a group of specialists will get involved in, and share responsibilities and decisions for a patient's care. It has been found that 65 or more significant decision points will be required across disciplines for the diagnosis and treatment of breast cancer [3]. Therefore, it is important to provide the clinical decision support that can effectively retrieve up-to-date clinical knowledge, match the knowledge against patient data and interpret implication, and assist clinicians to make the best decisions in compliance with the evidence. Representation and execution of clinical knowledge in formal guideline languages towards decision support is a widely recognised approach

© Springer International Publishing AG 2016
X. Yin et al. (Eds.): HIS 2016, LNCS 10038, pp. 9–21, 2016.
DOI: 10.1007/978-3-319-48335-1_2

but enactment of guidelines today is typically centrally orchestrated. This is inconsistent with real life situations as specialists work in quite ad hoc ways, dynamic in the nature of participation and collaboration, and over a flexible time period and space scope. Hence, a distributed decision support architecture is required to cope the challenges raised by complex diseases such as breast cancer, with the growing specialisation and ever increasing inter-relation in medicine today.

To this end, we work closely with the team from Oxford University where the widely regarded guideline language of PRO*forma* has been originally established and engaged in decision support for the past thirty years. A distributed decision support architecture is proposed in this paper to fit today's environment, and it will be based on the agent technology with many advantages in applying to medicine [4].

2   The Background of Guideline Languages and PRO*forma*

Evidence-Based Medicine promotes conscious and explicit use of best evidence in making clinical decisions [5]. Evidence may be gained from rigorous scientific studies and after evaluation, the strongest evidence will be used to design and develop clinical guidelines that apply to populations: "systematically developed statements to assist practitioners and patient to make decisions about appropriate health care for specific circumstances" [6]. In the UK, the National Institute for Health and Clinical Excellence (NICE) provides national clinical guidelines, e.g. [2, 11] for breast cancer, enabling timely translation of research findings into health and economic benefits. However, compliance with guidelines in practice leaves much to be desired, due to unawareness of such guidelines by clinicians and lack of robust implementation.

For these reasons, clinical guidelines are computerised and formally represented from conventional paper-based format, whereas patient symptoms and signs are matched with guidelines, candidate clinical options can be offered and evaluated, patient-specific advices generated, and direct links provided to the supporting evidence as part of the advices. This will raise the quality of care, as decision-making is in consistency with published and peer-reviewed evidence. Representation of guidelines using formal guideline representation languages is growing, including Arden Syntax [7], Guideline Interchange Format (GLIF) [8], PRO*forma* [9, 10] and so on.

PRO*forma* is a computer-executable clinical guideline and process representation language, developed at Cancer Research UK. The language provides a small number of generic task classes for composing into clinical task networks: An *Enquiry* is a task for acquiring information from a source (users, local records, remote systems, etc.). A *Decision* is any kind of choice between several options (diagnosis, risk classification, treatment selection, etc.). An *Action* is any kind of operation that will effect some change to the external world (administration of an injection or a prescribing). A *Plan* is a "container" for any number of tasks of any type, including other plans, usually in a specific order. On completion of modelling PRO*forma* tasks for a guideline, an application will be enacted by an engine. It has web contents dynamically generated on interface during the execution of tasks, i.e. forms for requesting information, groups of checkboxes or radio-buttons for choosing among decision candidates, and declaration about clinical procedures to be carried out. PRO*forma*'s simple task model has proved to be capable of modelling a range of clinical processes and decisions, and a wide range of applications have been developed over the past thirty years (see [10] for detailed syntax and semantics of the language and www.openclinical.net for use cases).

3 Triple Assessment for Breast Cancer

Triple Assessment is a common procedure in the National Health Service of UK for women suspected with breast cancer and referred to specialised breast units. Patients may be presented by their GPs [11] or following breast screening in the case of women aged between 50 and 70 who are invited for screening mammography every 3 years, through the NHS Breast Screening Programme (NHSBSP) in England [12] or the Breast Test Wales Screening Programme (BTWSP) in Wales. In both situations, it is best practice to carry out, in the breast unit, a "same day" clinic for evaluating the grade and spread of the cancer, if any, or a "*triple*" assessment:

1. Clinical and genetic risk assessment,
2. Imaging assessment by mammography or ultrasound (which radiological investigations to perform),
3. Pathology assessment by core biopsy, fine needle aspiration, or skin biopsy (which pathological investigations to perform).

An optimum way needs to be selected to manage the patient based on examination, imaging and pathology results [13], and when these are considered together, the diagnostic accuracy can exceed 99 %. If a cancer diagnosis is confirmed, the patient may enter final treatment and management. A major part of the NICE Care Pathway [2] of "Early and locally advanced breast cancer overview" is shown in Fig. 1, where the triple assessment is a central component.

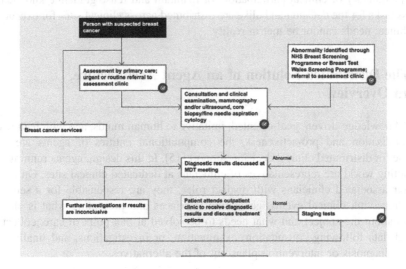

Fig. 1. A partial view of NICE Care Pathway for breast cancer

4   The Centralised Solution and Its Problems

The PRO*forma* representation of Triple Assessment guideline is presented in Fig. 2. It can be edited via a toolset, and saved to a single guideline file for central interpretation and execution via an engine.

In the specification, a "top level" plan is defined as a container for all tasks, starting from an '*examination*', an Enquiry type of task responsible for gathering relevant clinical examination information and genetic risk assessment. This is followed, when any abnormality is revealed, by a '*radiology_ decision*', a Decision type of task that determines which is the right mode of imaging for this patient. Three candidates, "do a mammogram of both breasts", "do an ultrasound of the affected area" and "do neither" are available for selection. After reasoning and recommendation, and a user confirmation, either a '*mammography_enquiry*' or '*ultrasound_enquiry*' may run to collect data regarding the imaging test result. The process continues with a '*biopsy_ decision*', that determines which is the right mode of biopsy among four candidates of "ultrasound/mammogram/freehand guided core biopsy", "ultrasound/mammogram/ freehand guided fine needle aspiration", "skin biopsy", and "no biopsy". A biopsy method will be selected and later performed, and data regarding the test result collected (on examination of the tissue sent to pathologist). Finally, a '*management_decision*' will run and consider all of three test results, referring the patient to other speciality/geneticist, entering the patient to a multidisciplinary meeting with high/low suspicion of cancer for surgery and/or adjuvant therapy, or into a high-risk follow-up protocol.

In this single specification, "Decision" components for distinctive expertises have been intertwined, along with data definition, referencing, and so on. "Enquiry" components for data gathering at various sites have also been mixed up. It will be hard, at the moment, to separate decision logic from other abstractions of data or computation, clarify boundary of clinical participation, or maintain and reuse guideline knowledge. Unless tasks for the decision and alike are distributed across clinical sites for execution, the clinical needs cannot be met in reality.

5   The Distributed Solution of an Agent Architecture, an Overview

Being knowledge-driven, goal-oriented, imitative to human minds, and with features of decentralisation and pro-activeness, the computational entities of agents are very suitable for distributed clinical decision support [15]. In this design, agents running in a computing world are representatives of clinicians at dedicated clinical sites. On behalf of their associated clinicians with distinct roles, they are responsible for a series of tasks: receiving clinical events, generating interfaces and presenting what is already known about the subject and what needs to be solved at that point of care, collecting clinical data following consultation, examination, or investigations, and finally suggesting diagnosis or intervention plans out of the alternatives.

```
/** PROforma (plain text) version 1.7.0 **/
metadata  :: ' ' ;
title :: 'triple_assessment' ; ......
data  :: 'patient_age' ;
     type :: integer ;
     caption :: 'What is the patient\'s age?' ;
end data.
data  :: 'patient_latestExamination_nippleDischarge' ;
     type :: text ;
     caption :: 'Does the patient have nipple discharge?' ;
     range ::"no","yes";
end data.
......
plan  :: 'triple_assessment' ;
     component :: 'examination' ;
     component :: 'further_investigation_decision' ;
          schedule_constraint :: completed('examination') ;
     component :: 'radiology_decision' ;
          schedule_constraint :: completed('further_investigation_decision') ;
     component :: 'ultrasound_enquiry' ;
          schedule_constraint :: completed('radiology_decision') ;
     component :: 'mammography_enquiry' ;
          schedule_constraint :: completed('radiology_decision') ;
     component :: 'biopsy_decision' ;
          schedule_constraint :: completed('ultrasound_enquiry') ;
          schedule_constraint :: completed('mammography_enquiry') ;
     component :: 'manage_patient_plan' ;
          schedule_constraint :: completed('biopsy_decision') ;
     component :: 'discharge_plan' ;
          schedule_constraint :: completed('further_investigation_decision') ;
......
plan  :: 'manage_patient_plan' ;
precondition :: result_of(further_investigation_decision) = manage_patient
or result_of(further_investigation_decision) = do_further_investigations;
     component :: 'treatment_decision' ;
     component :: 'management_decision' ;
          schedule_constraint :: completed('treatment_decision') ;
     component :: 'refer_to_other_speciality' ;
          schedule_constraint :: completed('management_decision') ;
     component :: 'corrective_surgery' ;
          schedule_constraint :: completed('management_decision') ;
     component :: 'give_drugs_action' ;
          schedule_constraint :: completed('management_decision') ;
     component :: 'follow_up' ;
          schedule_constraint :: completed('management_decision') ;
     component :: 'inform_gp' ;
          schedule_constraint :: completed('management_decision') ;
......
end plan.
......
plan  :: 'discharge_plan' ;
     precondition ::result_of(further_investigation_decision) = discharge;
     component :: 'reassure_and_discharge' ;
     component :: 'inform_gp' ;
end plan.
```

Fig. 2. The PROforma specification for Triple Assessment (the "orchestration" mode)

At runtime, collaborative sites will maintain their decision process, logic, and autonomy. Agents will retrieve the decision support knowledge executable to them, and share among themselves investigation results or decision outcomes by message passing. A number of common services such as data referencing, computation, and deduction will also be established. They can facilitate agents across multidisciplinary sites to be able to share the same consistent understanding of knowledge structure at design time, and draw up concrete clinical data and decisions at runtime, but are out of the scope of this paper and not detailed further. Previously, PRO*forma* composes clinical tasks such as enquiries, decisions, and actions into clinical decision processes for breast cancer, under a centralised or "orchestration" execution control. That model is reorganised into a set of interaction among separate agents in a distributed or "choreography" manner, agent tasks being temporally scheduled and activated under sequential or conditional circumstances, as shown in Fig. 3.

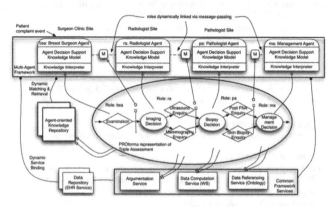

Fig. 3. The distributed architecture for breast cancer (the "choreography" mode)

The most prominent notions that need to be raised in this design may be a *Goal*, being a desired state to which a subject seeks to reach from the current state; an agent *Architecture*, where often a goal cannot be reached directly in one go by the subject alone, instead others may join and this forms an architecture; and a *Plan*, which will be drawn up by an individual agent in executing decision logic, sharing the decision result in the architecture, and coordinate among agents towards their shared goal.

The centralised decision model of PRO*forma* and the distributed agent decision model are shown side by side in Fig. 4. In the upper part, four types of tasks of PRO*forma* as mentioned in Sect. 2 are present. They are used for the composition of task-networks and server the centralised decision model. Here two cognitive state-transition cycles specify how a decision may be made prior to its implied action carried out [9]. Each round of decision-making runs iteratively and separately, with no explicit connection between them. In the lower part, two cycles are present in the distributed model as well, where an agent architecture is made up (cycle in blue) prior to each agent constructing its own plan (cycle in green). The agent architecture is made up in such a way that its corresponding goal reflects what needs to be addressed (start-up by an event in line a), collectively by multiple agents and which decomposes and assigns tasks to individual agents (end-up in plans in line b). The decomposition of a goal into assignable sub-goals makes the distributed decision architecture (line c), and the construction, processing, and execution of plans makes individual agent decisions (line d). The reference model of distributed decision-making shown in Fig. 4 will be further illustrated of its application to Triple Assessment in the next section as follows: goal-decomposition (Sect. 6.1), agent planning (Sect. 6.2), agent argumentation (Sect. 6.3), and towards implementation (Sect. 6.4).

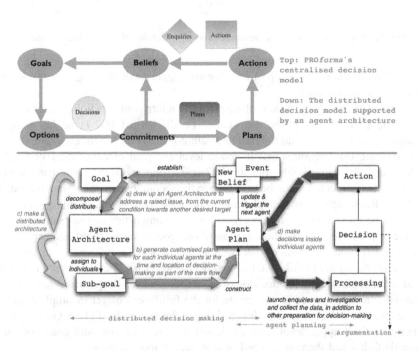

Fig. 4. The original centralised decision model and the distributed agent decision model (Color figure online)

6   Goal-Decomposition, Agent Planning, and Argumentation

6.1   The Goal-Decomposition Structure

The generic process of goal-decomposition for making the distributed decision architecture in Fig. 4 is applied here to the Triple Assessment scenario. A goal-decomposition tree structure is constructed after several decomposition iterations, with its top-level goal as root at top right through atomic sub-goals as leaves at bottom, shown in the left hand side of Fig. 5. Also, the generic process of constructing plans is applied several times and three of which are shown with concrete contents filled up in the right hand side of Fig. 5. A plan is central to an agent in capturing a sequential task workflow and responsible for achieving a sub-goal in a hierarchical goal-decomposition

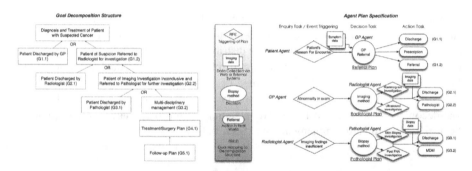

Fig. 5. A goal-decomposition structure (and its matching plans) for breast cancer

structure and ultimately, a group of collaborative agents will plan together for accomplishing the top-level goal.

In the example, after a patient of suspicion is referred to a radiologist for investigation (sub-goal of G1.2), she may either be discharged (G2.1) or her imaging investigation inconclusive and referred to a pathologist for further investigation (G2.2). Accomplishing G1.2 requires that its lower level sub-goal of either G2.1 or G2.2 is satisfied (and the same holds true to G2.2, G3.2 and so forth). This part of goal structure with distinct tree branches can map to the second plan in the right hand side of Fig. 5, the Radiologist Agent employing an imaging method and deciding whether a patient can be ruled out of breast cancer or not and taking actions correspondingly. The outcome of plan execution or the selection of one goal branch against another not just guides the behaviour or action of this agent alone but also has influence over the agent architecture. As for the radiologist, the goal-decomposition suffices at level three of the tree structure regarding to one decision or level four (or even deeper later) to the other, additional agents may need to participate for the fulfillment of yet incomplete goal in the latter occasion. As opposed to that, arriving at the leaf node of G1.1, G2.1, or G3.1 implies that their upper level (and top-level) goal is achieved (sub-goals turn into actionable tasks) and there is no need of introducing more agents.

6.2   The Agent Planning Rules

The very fundamental structure of an Agent Plan in Fig. 5 includes an Event triggering component responsible for cross-site communication, a Decision component, and an Action component with recommended clinical interventions as a result. The Plan structure is compliant with the design principle of clinical decision support that customised clinical plans and actions need to be generated by matching generic guidelines against current patient-specific conditions [14]. The triplet structure can be extended and termed as **Agent Planning Rules** shown in Fig. 6, by making the plan execution context (its Goal) explicit and hiding away the low-level computational details (its Processing) in this abstraction. An agent may maintain high-level decision logic with regard to up-to-date clinical knowledge and meet upcoming needs, as soon as its Planning Rules (re-)configured. This will permit the same agent to use whatever local

Agent Planning Rules: {*Event, (Sub-)Goal, Processing, Decision, Action*}

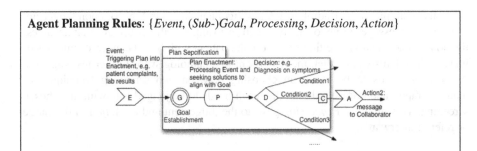

Event (*When* the Plan will be activated): Update the current state held towards the patient or environment, e.g. patient complaint, arrival of lab/exam result from other agents or systems;

Goal (*What* needs to be achieved): The state intended to bring about to patient or environment, e.g. give a diagnosis or treatment, or produce some intermediate results;

Processing (*How* can this be achieved): Given what is known (Event) and what needs to be established (Goal), collect and process whatever data required for Decision;

Decision (*Why* one of several alternatives is selected): Choose between different decision options, e.g. lab tests, diagnosis, prescribing or treatment plans;

Action (*What* will be done as a consequence and Who will join next): Take a clinical exam, injection, prescribing, referral of patient, or update a belief about diagnosis and so on.

Fig. 6. The scheme of Agent Planning Rules

resources available to solve different problems in participating different agent teams with different goals, but yet behave in a uniformly structured manner. This can offer us better maintainability, execute-ability, and separation of concerns.

Overall, the aimed agent decision architecture is event-driven and the dynamic matching, interpretation, and execution of **Agent Planning Rules** constitute the behaviour of individuals and the group, as follows:

(1) On receipt of a clinical **Event** (*When*), an agent matches it against its subscribed Planning Rules to find the appropriate one to deal with this, and populates this generic Planning Rule with specific situation data extracted from the message, which may indicate new patient data, lab or exam results available from another agent, etc.;

(2) The agent updates its current state about the environment, which causes it to establish a new **Goal** (*What*);

(3) Taking into account what is already known about the patient and what needs to be established by the Goal, the agent launches enquires about patient symptom, lab investigation and whatever data is missing prior to a decision being concluded and after certain computation and deduction, together structured as a **Processing** (*How*);

(4) A **Decision** (*Why*) can then be made: among a set of optional decision branches, each having a pre-condition for choosing this branch and an Action as post-condition of committing to it, the optimum one will be recommended with supporting evidence;

(5) An **Action** (*What*) will be committed eventually, either automatically or with user authorisation. In many cases this includes the passing of a message to the next agent, moving towards collaborative decision-making and progressing along care pathway.

In the example of the Radiologist Agent (its Plan shown in Fig. 5), upon the receipt of an *Event* message on abnormality found in exam, it will set up an imaging investigation to reach a *Goal* of either ruling out the patient with breast cancer, or findings of imaging inconclusive and then the result sent to a pathologist for further investigation. A *Decision* needs to be made on choosing between two screening techniques of mammography and ultrasound, and the result needs to be judged following the chosen screening. This involves *Processing* prior to the judgement and an *Action* of discharge or referral afterwards.

6.3   The Agent Argumentation Rules

In Agent Planning Rules, a decision may lead to different actions in different circumstances, thus the selection of a diagnosis, treatment, or care pathway among many choices. **Agent Argumentation Rules** can be linked to this decision structure in order to support reasoning. They represent declarative logic relationship between clinical

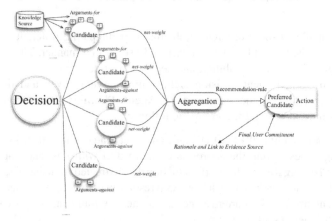

Agent Argumentation Rules: {*Decision, Candidates (arguments-for* weight, *arguments-against* weight), *Recommendation-rule, Action* Preferred-Candidate}

Decision: One includes several options (no decision needs to be made if only one persists) called candidates, among which one must be chosen;

Candidate: Each one of these can support the accomplishment of the Goal of decision-making, arguments either in support for or against every candidate need to be established, it should be from a recognised knowledgebase that the decision options available and arguments in relation with them are provided;

Argument (for or against): It offers the rationale about why a Candidate should be chosen or not, usually including a Condition being evaluated as true, a Type being support-for or support-against, and an assigned Weight to claim the strength or importance of the evidence;

Recommendation-rule: It recommends one of the options as a Preferred Candidate, on the basis of aggregating the net-support that each option acquires, this involves a process of evaluating each of these arguments (for or against) as true or false and calculating weights;

Action: An Action associated with the Preferred Candidate will be carried out eventually, it may be a clinical treatment, an investigation, or the update of a belief on a diagnosis.

Fig. 7. The scheme of Agent Argumentation Rules

symptoms or other findings as premise, and judgment of arguments in support for or against decision candidates as consequence, shown in Fig. 7.

In the example of Radiologist Agent, a **Decision** needs to be made on the use of an imaging method for investigation, with two **Candidates** available: *Candidate 1* "Do a mammogram of both breasts" and *Candidate 2* "Do an ultrasound of the affected area". The rational in deciding between them is provided by guidelines and evidence shows that, **Arguments** that support *Candidate 1* include if the patient has been assessed as being at medium or high genetic risk and is over 30 years old, if she has a nipple inversion, axillary lymph node, non-cyclical breast pain, or localised breast nodularity, among others; **Arguments** against *Candidate 1* include if the patient is pregnant, if she is younger than 35 years old, among others. Arguments for or against *Candidate 2* can be established likewise with corresponding weights. A Preferred Candidate will then be provided following a **Recommendation-rule**, as the satisfaction of arguments can be evaluated and the net-support of each candidate calculated and aggregated, not detailed in this paper. An **Action** of discharging the patient or referring her to a pathologist will be carried out as the eventual outcome.

```
G := G₀ // the top-level goal
G_list := decompose(G)
while not empty(G_list) do
    get next G_i from G_list
    // find all agents which are able and willing to play the associated role
    A_list := callForParticipation(matchRole(G_i))
    if not empty(A_list) then
        // select a potential agent from the list
        Agent_i := select(A_list)
        // find from knowledgebase all the candidates that can satisfy the sub-goal
        O_list := options(satisfy(KB, post-condition(G_i)))
        O_ordered-list := argumentation(O_list) // invoke the argumentation and order the options
        O_i := select(O_ordered-list) // get the best possible option for now
        P_i := plan(Agent_i, O_i)
        // re-plan if the sub-goal cannot be satisfied
        while not succeeded(P_i) do
                execute(P_i)
                S_i := belief(Agent_i)
                // check if the sub-goal succeeds after executing the chosen plan
                if satisfy(S_i, post-condition(G_i)) then
                        succeeded(P_i)
                        belief(Agent_{i+1}, S_i) // share the current patient data and decisions
                        pre-condition(G_{i+1}) := post-condition(G_i) // link the goal states
                else
                        O_i := select-next(O_ordered-list) // get the next best possible option
                        P_i := plan(Agent_i, O_i) // re-plan for this agent
                end-if
        end-while
    end-if
end-while
```

Fig. 8. An algorithm for goal-decomposition, agent planning and argumentation

6.4   Towards Implementation of the Distributed Agent Decision Architecture

Upon the completion of executing **Agent Argumentation Rule** on two investigation methods and the imaging result judged to be suspicious, relevant data will be sent to a pathologist on patient referral. It completes the **Agent Planning Rule** of this agent and indicates a step further to the goal. Interactive interfaces between agents and their assisting clinicians will be activated at radiologist site and others, and thus support provided for decision-making in the distributed environment as shown in Fig. 3. An algorithm for implementing the overall architecture is shown in Fig. 8.

7   Discussion and Conclusions

In this paper, an agent-oriented decision support architecture is put forward to drive distributed decision-making for breast cancer. The work reviews and addresses the issues raised by the centralised approach of PRO*forma* and a generic distributed solution is provided: (1) goal-decomposition structure supports the shaping of the agent decision architecture and the elaboration of plans; (2) agent planning rules support individual decision-making with a goal-achieving capability and an agent-executable structure; and (3) agent argumentation rules further support reasoning among decision options and provide a mechanism for recommending a preferred option, being an appropriate diagnostic test, a treatment option, or a particular care pathway. The work builds on top of our previous work [15] and the use of the Triple Assessment of breast cancer scenario illustrates the shift from a centralised decision-making solution to a distributed one. However, the approach is not limited just to this particular problem. Instead, we are working on this generic and versatile approach and applying it to a wider range of clinical guideline knowledgebase across medicine and will make it more powerful for distributed decision support by agents.

Acknowledgment. This work is supported by National Natural Science Foundation of China (61202101) & Dept. of Health on Data Exchange Standard for Hubei Provincial Care Platform.

References

1. NHS North of England Cancer Network: Breast Cancer Clinical Guidelines, p. 4 (2011)
2. National Institute for Clinical Excellence: Healthcare services for breast cancer (2002)
3. Patkar, V., et al.: Evidence-based guidelines and decision support services: a discussion and evaluation in triple assessment of suspected breast cancer. Br. J. Cancer **95**(11), 1490–1496 (2006)
4. Moreno, A., Nealon, J.L. (eds.): Application of Software Agent Technology in the Health Care Domain. Birkhäuser, Switzerland (2003)
5. Sackett, D.L., Rosenberg, W.M.C., Gray, J.A.M., Haynes, R.B., Richardson, W.S.: Evidence based medicine: what it is and what it isn't. BMJ **312**, 71 (1996)

6. Field, M.J., Lohr, K.N. (eds.): Clinical Practice Guidelines: Directions for a New Program. Institute of Medicine. National Academy Press, Washington, DC (1990)
7. Hripcsak, G., Ludemann, P., Pruor, T.A., Wigertz, O.B., Clayton, P.B.: Rationale for the Arden syntax. Comput. Biomed. Res. **27**(4), 291–324 (1994)
8. Peleg, M., et al.: GLIF3: the evolution of a guideline representation format. In: Proceedings of the AMIA Symposium, pp. 645–649 (2000)
9. Fox, J., Das, S.: Safe and Sound: Artificial Intelligence in Hazardous Applications. Jointly published by the AAAI, Menlo Park, CA, MIT Press, Cambridge Mass (2000)
10. Sutton, D.R., Fox, J.: The syntax and semantics of the PRO*forma* guideline modeling language. J. Am. Med. Inf. Assoc. **10**(5), 433–443 (2003)
11. National Institute for Health and Clinical Excellence (NICE): Referral guidelines for suspected cancer (CG27), p. 12 (2011)
12. NHS Cancer Screening Programmes: Non-operative diagnostic procedures and reporting in breast cancer screening (NHSBSP Publication No 50) (2001)
13. Royal College of Surgeons of England: Guidelines for the management of symptomatic breast disease (BASO). Eur. J. Surg. Oncol. **3**(1), S1–S21 (2005). Elsevier
14. Kawamoto, K., Houlihan, C.A., Balas, E.A., Lobach, D.F.: Improving clinical practice using clinical decision support systems: a systematic review of trials to identify features critical to success. BMJ **330**, 765 (2005)
15. Xiao, L., Fox, J., Zhu, H.: An agent-oriented approach to support multidisciplinary care decisions. In: Proceedings of the 3rd Eastern European Regional Conference on the Engineering of Computer Based Systems (ECBS 2013), pp. 8–17. IEEE (2013)

Improved GrabCut for Human Brain Computerized Tomography Image Segmentation

Zhihua Ji[1,2], Shaode Yu[1,3(✉)], Shibin Wu[1,3], Yaoqin Xie[1], and Fashun Yang[2]

[1] Shenzhen Institutes of Advanced Technology,
Chinese Academy of Sciences, Shenzhen, China
{zh.ji,sd.yu,sb.wu,yq.xie}@siat.ac.cn
[2] Academy of Big Data and Information Engineering,
Guizhou University, Guiyang, China
fashun@126.com
[3] Shenzhen College of Advanced Technology,
University of Chinese Academy of Sciences, Shenzhen 518055, China
http://www.siat.ac.cn

Abstract. In this paper, we modified GrabCut for gray-scale slice-stacked medical image segmentation. First, GrabCut was extended from planar to volume image processing. Second, we simplified manual interaction by drawing a polygon for one volume instead of a rectangle. After that, twenty human brain computerized tomography images were analyzed. Experimental results show that the modified algorithm is simple and fast, and enhances segmentation accuracy compared with the confidence connection algorithm. Moreover, the algorithm is reproducible with respect to different users and consequently it can release physicians from this kind of time-consuming and laborious tasks. In addition, this method can be used for other types of medical volume image segmentation.

Keywords: Image segmentation · Computerized tomography · GrabCut

1 Introduction

Medical image segmentation is the basis for image analysis, disease diagnosis, treatment planning and image guided radiation therapy [1–6]. Manual segmentation is feasible but with very low efficiency. In particular, it may introduce subjective bias [7]. Semi-automated methods can incorporate prior knowledge for higher accuracy, but it is impractical in large-scale experiments [8,9]. A large number of automated image segmentation methods have been proposed [10–12]. However, most algorithms suffer from noise, parameter tuning, initialization or heavy computing complexity [10].

In theory, image segmentation can be expressed as an energy minimization problem. It aims to portion the whole image into several sub-graphs and achieves

X. Yin et al. (Eds.): HIS 2016, LNCS 10038, pp. 22–30, 2016.
DOI: 10.1007/978-3-319-48335-1_3

a minimum value of the cost function. Max-flow min-cut algorithms well handles this kind of problems. Boykov *et al.* proposed GraphCut algorithm [13] and introduced how to construct the graph and function of energy minimization. Many related methods have been proposed [14–18], while GrabCut distinguishes itself from reduced manual interaction and improved segmentation results [15]. Subsequently, GrabCut is mainly modified to address segmentation of videos [19–22]. Technically, three-dimension (3D) GrabCut has also been proposed. [23] proposed it for interactive foreground extraction and 3D scene reconstruction, while [24] developed for real-time applications and has no systematical evaluation. In this paper, the goal is to extend GrabCut from planar space to 3D space and handles gray-scale slice-stacked medical images. Firstly, GrabCut was extended from planar to volume image processing. Second, we simplified manual interaction by drawing a polygon for one volume instead of a rectangle. After that, twenty human brain computerized tomography images were analyzed.

The remaining of this paper is organized as follows. Section 2 describes the basic methods and the improved algorithm. Section 3 presents experimental results of brain volumes, time cost and the performance of the proposed algorithm. In the end, we will summarize this paper in Sect. 4.

2   Methods and Materials

2.1   GrabCut

GrabCut is an iterative segmentation technique. It draws a rectangle around the object and uses the textural and boundary information for image segmentation. GrabCut expresses an image with an undirected graph $G=<V, E>$, where V is the vertex set and E is the edge set. Specially, the graph has two more vertexes. One is s named source point and another one is t named sink point.

Figure 1 illustrates the s-t graph of an image. Every pixel corresponds to a vertex of the graph. In addition, s and t are included in the graph. Figure 1 contains two kinds of edges, solid lines named n-links and dotted lines named t-links. n-links represent the edges between two adjacent ordinary vertexes and t-links represent the edges between s (or t) and ordinary vertexes. Each edge with weight shows the similarities between the two vertexes of the edge. The purpose of GrabCut is to find a set of edges, the sum of weights of which is minimum, to make the sub-graph including s and the sub-graph including t unconnected.

The GrabCut methold includes two GMMs, one for the background and one for the foreground. The energy function to be minimized is shown in Eq. 1, in which $U(\alpha, k, \theta, z)$ is region energy and $V(\alpha, z)$ is boundary energy.

$$E(\alpha, k, \theta, z) = U(\alpha, k, \theta, z) + V(\alpha, z) \tag{1}$$

Where K is the number of Gaussian components in a GMM, typically K equals to 5. One component either from the background or foreground model, according as $\alpha = 0$ or 1. The parameters of the model are

$$\theta = \{\pi(\alpha, k), \mu(\alpha, k), \Sigma(\alpha, k)\} \tag{2}$$

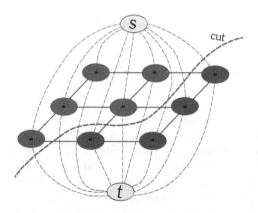

Fig. 1. *s-t* Graph. Image segmentation is transferred to find a cut (blue dotted line) to separate the foreground (red rounds) and the background (green rounds). (Color figure online)

$U(\alpha, k, \theta, z)$ corresponds to weights between connected nodes (n-links). How to calculate the weights between pixel m and n is expressed in Eq. 3,

$$N(m,n) = k * e^{-\beta||z_m - z_n||^2} \tag{3}$$

where $||z_m - z_n||$ is the Euclidean distance in color space, k is set 50 [27], while β is computed as in Eq. 4.

$$\beta = (2 < ||z_m - z_n||^2 >)^{-1} \tag{4}$$

$V(\alpha, z)$ corresponds to weights between nodes and special nodes (t-links). Shown in Fig. 1, each pixel has a t-link connected with the background (T_b) and with the foreground (T_f). The user marks the region of interest (ROI) with rectangular. Pixels inside ROI are unknown and outside are background. In order to know each pixel inside the rectangular belong to foreground or background, we should calculate the value of its label. Suppose that the t-link between each pixel and source node is T_1 and the t-link between each pixel and sink node is T_2. If one pixel belongs to foreground, then $T_1 = K_{max}$ and $T_2 = 0$, else $T_1 = 0$ and $T_2 = K_{max}$. K_{max} is the maximum possible weight of every edge. If one pixel is unknown, we should compute its probability using Gaussian mixture model (GMM) as shown in Eq. 5,

$$P(m) = -log \sum_{i=1}^{k} P(m,i) \tag{5}$$

$P(m,i)$ is the probability that one pixel belongs to the ith Gaussian component.

2.2   Proposed Algorithm

The contributions of this paper are as following. On the one hand, it is implemented toward 3D image processing, namely, it extends the *s-t* graph from plain to stereogram. On the other hand, users manually initialize the potential foreground with a polygon instead of a rectangle. In practice, it is found that drawing a rectangle is not convenient when the object has an irregular boundary. So users only need to draw several points outside the boundary of the object in one slice and the algorithm connects the points to produce a polygon as the ROI automatically. Meanwhile, the modified algorithm is verified on twenty brain volumes and the implemented algorithm is ready for public access.

After manual initialization, nodes inside ROI are possible foreground and nodes outside ROI are background. Then, the proposed algorithm forms a flow network and every voxel is one node of the network. Once the graph is built, the whole graph is isolated into two unconnected sub-graph using max-flow/min-cut. If necessary, additional edition can be involved.

2.3 Evaluation Criterion

Segmentation accuracy is validated from DICE coefficient which measures brain overlapping between the ground truth (G) and the segmentation result (S). It is defined as below.

$$DICE = 2 \times \frac{|G \cap S|}{|G| + |S|}. \tag{6}$$

where $| \cdot |$ indicates volume computed as the number of voxels. Besides, time consumption (tc) to each image slice is also concerned, $tc = \frac{1}{n}\sum_{i=1}^{n} tc_i$. Where tc_i is the time consumption of the ith slice and n is the slice number of the three-dimension medical image.

2.4 Experiment Design

Twenty brain volumes are collected, which are from personal data set. The physical resolution is $[0.5,\ 0.5,\ 3.0]\,mm^3$. The proposed algorithm is systematically compared with the confidence connection algorithm (CCA) [25]. In addition, the reproducibility of the proposed algorithm was tested and initialized from three different users.

All codes are implemented on VS2010, and running on a workstation with 4 Intel(R) Cores(TM) of 3.70 GHz and 8 GB RAM. Involved third-party softwares are OpenCV, VTK and ITK.

3   Results and Discussion

3.1 Rectangle Vs. Polygon

One image slice is initialized with a rectangle and a polygon respectively, and corresponding segmentation results are shown in Fig. 2. It is found that drawing a polygon is much easier than drawing a rectangle, because a polygon can be delineated closer to the object boundary. In addition, the segmentation result initialized with a polygon is more precise and smooth than with a rectangle.

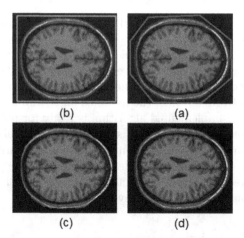

(b)   (a)

(c)   (d)

Fig. 2. Algorithm initialization by drawing a rectangle and a polygon. (a) the original brain image, (b) the original brain image, (c) Brain segmentation result initialized with rectangle, and (d) Brain segmentation result initialized with polygon.

Therefore, in further analysis, we suggest drawing a polygon instead of a rectangle to initialize the proposed segmentation algorithm. We can see that drawing a polygon is more convenient and gets a more accurate segmentation result.

3.2 Performance Comparison

Two methods are compared based on DICE and time consumption as shown in Fig. 3. From DICE coefficient, it is found that GC is about 8 % higher than CCA. The average DICE of GC is 0.98 and CCA is 0.90. This is mainly because that CT brain images are with high visual quality and tissue contrast. In addition, from time cost, GC takes half the time of CCA for one slice segmentation and is more efficient. The average time of GC is 3.17 s and CCA is 6.41 s.

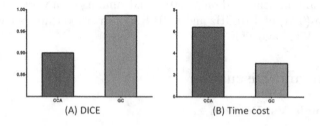

(A) DICE   (B) Time cost

Fig. 3. Performance comparison on CT brain image segmentation.

3.3 Visual Comparison

Figure 4 shows a representative for visual observation. (a) is the original image, (b) is the segmentation result by CCA and (c) is from GC. (d, e, f) are the third slice from (a, b, c), respectively. It is observed that there are artifacts or ghosting in the original image. After image segmentation, these artifacts are removed clearly by GC. However, it is also found that CCA causes holes in the brain region, particular these bright regions of skull and bones. On contrary, GC finishes this task more completely and effectively.

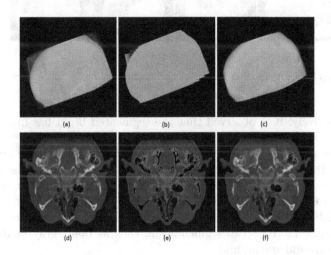

Fig. 4. The visualization of brain segmentation results. (a) is the original image, (b) is the segmentation result by CCA and (c) is from GC. (d, e, f) are the third slice from (a, b, c), respectively.

3.4 Algorithm's Reproducibility

All CT images are chosen for testing the reproductivity of proposed algorithm, and three users are involved. One is a ten years radiologist and the other two are common users.

Table 1 shows the accuracy (DICE) and time cost to each user. Statistical analysis is based on paired-t test. We found the p value is 0.196 between #1 and #2, 0.320 between #2 and #3, and 0.6250 between #1 and #3. All p values from paired t-test larger than 0.05 indicate that there is no significant difference between each two users. That means, the proposed algorithm is stable and reproducible in medical image segmentation with respect to any user if and only if he draws a correct polygon to initialize the incomplete labeling. Most importantly, this kind of reproducibility releases physicians from endless and laborious tasks of organ segmentation.

Figure 5 shows the segmentation results of one CT data set. (a) is the original brain volume and (b, c, d) are the brain segmentation result by user 1, user 2 and

Table 1. Segmentation accuracy and time cost to each user.

User	DICE	Time cost (seconds)
#1	0.952 ± 0.005	125.3 ± 7.92
#2	0.946 ± 0.007	127.8 ± 8.05
#3	0.950 ± 0.009	120.1 ± 8.23

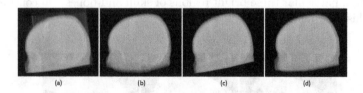

Fig. 5. Segmentation results of one brain volume by three users.

user 3 respectively. It is observed that the segmented brain has little artifacts and smooth surface.

The proposed algorithm is promising. However, there are several limitations. Technically, the number of components in GMMs is set as the default value and an optimal number might improve the performance. Meanwhile, automated segmentation is possible with proper algorithm deployment, such as automated incomplete labeling. In addition, it will be more interesting if the proposed algorithm can tackle more precise segmentation, such as bone, gray matter, white matter and cerebral spinal fluid.

4   Conclusion

GrabCut is modified for gray-scale slice-stacked medical image segmentation and the performance is validated from segmentation accuracy, real-time ability and reproducibility. Experiments have shown that the proposed algorithm is easy-to-use, high efficient, light computing and very stable. This algorithm can release physicians from laborious and tedious tasks of organ segmentation. In the next step, we may adjust this algorithm for precise tissue segmentation.

Acknowledgment. This work is supported by grants from National Natural Science Foundation of China (Grant No. 81501463), Guangdong Innovative Research Team Program (Grant No. 2011S013), National 863 Programs of China (Grant No. 2015AA043203), Shenzhen Fundamental Research Program (Grant Nos. JCYJ20140417113430726, JCYJ20140417113430665 and JCYJ201500731154850923) and Beijing Center for Mathematics and Information Interdisciplinary Sciences.

References

1. Dhawan, A.P.: Medical Image Analysis. Wiley, New York (2011)
2. Ezzell, G.A., Galvin, J.M., et al.: Guidance document on delivery, treatment planning, and clinical implementation of IMRT: report of the IMRT Subcommittee of the AAPM Radiation Therapy Committee. Med. Phys. **30**(8), 2089–2115 (2003)
3. Xing, L., Thorndyke, B., et al.: Overview of image-guided radiation therapy. Med. Dosim. **31**(2), 91–112 (2006)
4. Xie, Y., Djajaputra, D., et al.: Intrafractional motion of the prostate during hypofractionated radiotherapy. Int. J. Radiat. Oncol. Biol. Phys. **72**(1), 236–246 (2008)
5. Xie, Y., Chao, M., et al.: Feature-based rectal contour propagation from planning CT to cone beam CT. Med. Phys. **35**(10), 4450–4459 (2008)
6. Chao, M., Xie, Y., Xing, L.: Auto-propagation of contours for adaptive prostate radiation therapy. Phys. Med. Biol. **53**(17), 4533 (2008)
7. Khodr, Z.G., Sak, M.A., et al.: Determinants of the reliability of ultrasound tomography sound speed estimates as a surrogate for volumetric breast density. Med. Phys. **42**(10), 5671–5678 (2015)
8. Zhou, W., Xie, Y.: Interactive contour delineation and refinement in treatment planning of image-guided radiation therapy. J. Appl. Clin. Med. Phys. **15**(1), 4499 (2014)
9. Zhou, W., Xie, Y.: Interactive medical image segmentation using snake and multiscale curve editing. Comput. Math. Methods Med. **2013** (2013)
10. Pham, D.L., Xu, C., Prince, J.L.: Current methods in medical image segmentation. Annu. Rev. Biomed. Eng. **2**, 322–325 (2000)
11. Dirami, A., Hammouche, K., et al.: Fast multilevel thresholding for image segmentation through a multiphase level set method. Sig. Process. **93**(1), 139–153 (2013)
12. Cai, H., Yang, Z., et al.: A new iterative triclass thresholding technique in image segmentation. IEEE Trans. Image Process. **23**(3), 1038–1046 (2014)
13. Boykov, Y., Veksler, O., Zabih, R.: Fast approximate energy minimization via graph cuts. IEEE Trans. Pattern Anal. Mach. Intell. **1**(11), 1222–1239 (2001)
14. Boykov, Y.Y., Jolly, M.P.: Interactive graph cuts for optimal boundary and region segmentation of objects in N-D images. ICCV **2001**(1), 105–112 (2001)
15. Rother, C., Kolmogorov, V., Blake, A.: Grabcut: interactive foreground extraction using iterated graph cuts. ACM Trans. Graph. (TOG) **23**(3), 309–314 (2004)
16. Boykov, Y., Funka-Lea, G.: Graph cuts and efficient n-d image segmentation. Int. J. Comput. Vis. **70**(2), 109–131 (2006)
17. Yin, S., Zhao, X., Wang, W., Gong, M.: Efficient multilevel image segmentation through fuzzy entropy maximization and graph cut optimization. Pattern Recogn. **47**(9), 2894–2907 (2014)
18. Temoche, P., Carmona, R.: A volume segmentation approach based on GrabCut. CLEI Electron. J. **16**(2), 4–4 (2013)
19. Park, S., Yoo, J.H.: Human segmentation based on GrabCut in real-time video sequences. ICCE **2014**, 111–112 (2014)
20. Gao, Z., Shi, P., et al.: A mutual GrabCut method to solve co-segmentation. EURASIP J. Image Video Process. **2013**(1), 1–11 (2013)
21. Hernandez-Vela, A., Reyes, M., et al.: Grabcut-based human segmentation in video sequences. Sensors **12**(11), 15376–15393 (2012)

22. Li, J.G., Li, X.N., et al.: Application of GrabCut in human serially sectioned image segmentation. Comput. Technol. Develop. **21**(12), 246–249 (2011)
23. Meyer, G.P., Do, M.N.: 3D GrabCut: interactive foreground extraction for reconstructed 3D scenes. In: Eurographics Workshop on 3D Object Retrieval 2015, pp. 1–6. Eurographics Association (2015)
24. Ramirez, J., Temoche, P., Carmona, R.: A volume segmentation approach based on GrabCut. CLEI Electron. J. **16**(2), 4–4 (2013)
25. Piekos, T.: Confidence connected segmentation using ITK. Insight J. **2007** (2007)
26. Mortensen, E.N., Barrett, W.A.: Intelligent scissors for image composition. In: Proceedings of the 22nd Annual Conference on Computer Graphics and Interactive Techniques, pp. 191–198. ACM (1995)
27. Blake, A., Rother, C., Brown, M., Perez, P., Torr, P.: Interactive image segmentation using an adaptive GMMRF model. In: Pajdla, T., Matas, J. (eds.) ECCV 2004. LNCS, vol. 3021, pp. 428–441. Springer, Heidelberg (2004). doi:10.1007/978-3-540-24670-1_33

Web-Interface-Driven Development for Neuro3D, a Clinical Data Capture and Decision Support System for Deep Brain Stimulation

Shiqiang Tao[1], Benjamin L. Walter[2], Sisi Gu[3], and Guo-Qiang Zhang[1(✉)]

[1] Institute of Biomedical Informatics, University of Kentucky, Lexington, KY, USA
gq.zhang@uky.edu
[2] Department of Neurology, University Hospitals, Cleveland, OH, USA
[3] Department of Electrical Engineering and Computer Science,
Case Western Reserve University, Cleveland, OH, USA

Abstract. Parkinson's Disease is a common chronic neurological motor system disorder that affects more than 10 million people worldwide with no known cure. With Deep Brain Stimulation (DBS) emerging as one of the main treatments for Parkinson's Disease, the effective capture, retrieval, and analysis of data generated from DBS are important informatics challenges. To address these challenges, this paper presents the design and implementation of Neuro3D, a web-interfaced system for DBS data capture and management in the clinical setting. Neuro3D provides: (1) data capture interfaces with multiple data entry assistances and validations to improve both the data entry efficiency and the data quality; (2) intuitive data organization that mirrors the workflow of clinical operations; and (3) a novel data exploration as a basis for clinical decision support. Neuro3D accomplishes these utilizing an agile development strategy called Web-Interface-Driven Development (WIDD) to optimize the communication between software developers and domain experts. 36 distinct data forms consisting of 1109 discrete data elements are captured and managed in Neuro3D. Pilot deployment of Neuro3D in the Movement Disorders Center of the University Hospitals Neurological Institute in Cleveland captured clinical data for 236 patients, in a comprehensive and research-ready fashion beyond the scope of current EMR. Neuro3D fills an important void in terms of tools for capturing large-scale clinical neurology data to improve care and outcome for patients with Parkinson's disease.

1 Introduction

Parkinson's disease (PD) is one of the most common neurodegenerative disorders. It mainly affects the motor systems, caused by the loss of dopamine-producing brain cells. Primary symptoms of PD are tremor, rigidity, bradykinesia, or slowness of movement; and postural instability, or impaired balance and coordination [1]. According to the Parkinson's Disease Foundation [2], PD affects one million people in the United States and more than ten million worldwide.

© Springer International Publishing AG 2016
X. Yin et al. (Eds.): HIS 2016, LNCS 10038, pp. 31–42, 2016.
DOI: 10.1007/978-3-319-48335-1_4

Patients with PD are estimated to grow substantially in the next twenty years according to a project conducted in the five most populous Western Europe nations and the world's ten most populous nations [3].

PD can last for years or lifelong. At present, there is no cure for PD. Usually, patients affected by PD are given levodopa combined with carbidopa to relieve the symptoms. However, not all patients respond to medications and even when they do, there are side effects such as dyskinesias. Deep Brain Stimulation (DBS) is a treatment procedure for PD approved by the U.S. Food and Drug Administration (FDA). In DBS, electrodes are implanted into the patient brain, providing electric pulses to alleviate the symptoms of PD. DBS can reduce the need for levodopa and related medications, which in turn decreases the side effects [1].

In the past two decades, approximately 60,000 patients worldwide with PD have undergone DBS, with an annual accrual of 8000 to 10,000 new patients [4]. The success of DBS relies on the careful patient selection, precise surgery plan, and optimal programming of the stimulator device parameter settings [5]. Because of this, DBS generates large volumes of data. The accuracy, accessibility, legibility and processability of the large quantity of patient information associated with DBS and individual specific decision making can affect the quality of care and outcomes. No off-the-shelf digital tools exist to capture the electrophysiological data acquired for DBS, such as locations, stimulation variables, and associated therapeutic benefits and side effects for the implanted electrodes. An integrated system managing the entire lifecycle of DBS clinical data is needed.

This paper presents the design and implementation of a web-based, vendor-independent system, called Neurological Deep Data for DBS (Neuro3D), for capturing and managing clinical data for DBS. To address the challenges of the multitudes of data capturing points and multiple roles involved in a multi-stage process, the traditional waterfall software development model is inadequate to handle the combination of complexities in system architecture, data schema design, role-based access control, and usability. We developed a unique agile development process to address the complexity of development process: *Web-Interface-Driven Development (WIDD)*. WIDD allows domain experts and users to participate in every step of system development for Neuro3D. Neuro3D is designed to be integrated into the clinical workflow and mirror the actual DBS procedure. The system captures longitudinal clinical data in three stages: (1) pre-operative registration and assessments; (2) intra-operative surgical data acquisition; and (3) post-operative evaluation and adjustment.

Neuro3D integrates the data collected from all stages of the procedure, organizes data by clinical visits, reduces data management complexity, and ultimately improves the quality and efficiency of the entire clinical workflow.

2   Background

2.1   Parkinson's Disease Treatment

Medications are available for treating PD, such as levodopa, dopamine agonists and monoamine oxidase (MAO)-B inhibitors. They are widely used to alleviate the PD symptoms and reduce the risk of dyskinesia. For PD patients with a major depressive disorder, interpersonal psychotherapy proves to be a feasible treatment to improve depression symptoms [6]. However, despite the advances of pharmacotherapy and psychotherapy, there are drawbacks to each treatment options. The medications take effect initially, but after five years of treatment a majority of patients no longer benefit from pharmacotherapy and can even develop medication related motor complications [7, 8]. Psychotherapy is partially or completely ineffective for some patients [9]. Therefore, while treatment options are available for most patients, some PD patients are treatment-resistant and even unresponsive to both psychotherapy and pharmacotherapy [10].

2.2   Deep Brain Stimulation

Deep brain stimulation is an FDA approved neurosurgical treatment procedure appropriate for PD patients who cannot benefit from either pharmacotherapy or psychotherapy. It is a clinically proven successful technique with concomitant obsessive-compulsive disorder or treatment-resistant depression [11].

Figure 1 shows the workflow of DBS procedure and patient data generated at each step. First, patient demographic and registration information are recorded along with referring physician information. Afterward, PD rating scales and other medical information are captured to evaluate the DBS qualification. Following that, a multidisciplinary team consisting of movement disorders neurologists, functional neurosurgeons, and neuropsychologists holds a care conference to determine the applicability and optimal surgical plans regarding the DBS procedure. If qualified, a patient undergoes stereotactic imaging procedures such as MRI or CT to decide the target brain area to implant the micro-electrodes. During surgery, micro-electrodes are precisely implanted in some brain areas guided a combination of stereotactic and neuro-imaging techniques. A programmable subcutaneous external pacemaker is implanted in a patient's chest area. After surgery, programming sessions are scheduled and adjustments on the pacemaker are made with respect to electrode configuration, voltage amplitude, pulse width, and frequency to send electrical currents to the brain for the best outcomes. All benefits and adverse events are recorded to help the physicians make appropriate modifications and other decisions.

A DBS program consists of a combination of roles and cores, as shown in Table 1. In neurological and neurosurgical practices, people act in different roles such as Neurologist, Neurosurgeon, Neuropsychologist, Nurse, Fellow, and Resident.

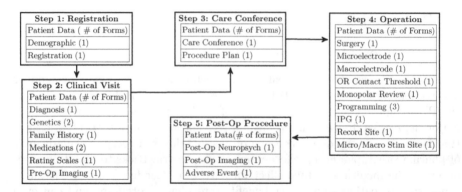

Fig. 1. Illustrative diagram of a typical DBS workflow.

Different cores manage different aspects of patient data. For example, administrative core records patient demographic information and registration information while surgery core stores surgery-related information like DBS leads and stimulation sites. People of different roles have different responsibilities and different data access levels. For the first time, Neuro3D formalizes and manages roles and cores using role-based access control (RBAC) [12] for DBS programs.

Table 1. The roles and cores of a typical DBS program.

Roles	Cores
Neurologist	Administrative Core
Neurosurgeon	Clinical Core
Neuropsychologist	Surgery Core
Nurse	Neuropsychological Core
Fellow	Imaging Core
Resident	Adverse Events Core

2.3   User Interface Design

User interface design is one of the most important and difficult software engineering problems. User interface directly connects the user and the system and defines how the user interacts with the system to accomplish certain tasks [13,14]. Because of the data complexity involved in DBS, user interface design is a critical component in the development of Neuro3D, which is the key motivation behind WIDD.

3   Methods

We implement Neuro3D following WIDD, which follows the model-view-controller (MVC) architectural pattern that enforces a separation between (also called business logic) from the input and presentation logic associated with a graphical user interface (GUI). With WIDD, our technical team collect system specifications and build Neuro3D as a flexible patient-data oriented system with built-in access control for users of multiple roles. In the following subsections, we describe the details about WIDD methodology and other best practices we used in the system design and implementation of Neuro3D.

3.1   Web Interface Driven Development

Building a clinical system requires software developers to understand the clinical operations before they can make design decisions. However, software developers usually have limited medical background and users of the system have limited understanding in software development. To address this communication gap, we propose the WIDD approach for the design and development of Neuro3D. As an illustration, Fig. 2 shows how Neuro3D follows WIDD in designing and construct-ing the forms for Unified Parkinson's Disease Rating Scale (UPDRS) [16], one of the most commonly used scales in the clinical study of PD. WIDD contains four general steps: (1) requirements elicitation; (2) interface construction and revision; (3) user review and feedback; and (4) implementation and deployment.

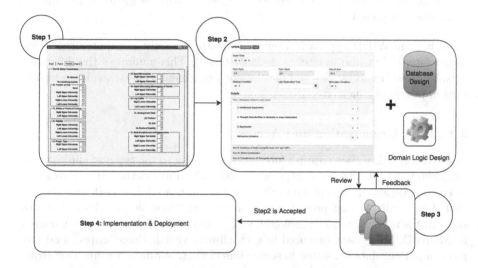

Fig. 2. Four steps of WIDD agile software development approach.

1. First, clinicians provide information about the functions they desire. The information is presented in multiple formats. For UPDRS, there are screen-shots (step 1 in Fig. 2) from existing EMR system, formal description form that defines the information recorded in UPDRS, and hand drawings from clinicians. The information covers the following aspects: (a) All fields that are captured in UPDRS; (b) The display label for each field and the value type for that field such as free text, selection list, or numerical value; and (c) Formula embedded in the form. UPDRS consists of four sections. Each section has a set of numerical fields. In addition to these fields, a weighted sum is computed for each section.
2. In step 2, initial web interfaces are created. The web interface has the ability to capture all fields in UPDRS, organize its four sections in accordion style, and calculate the sum value for each section automatically. As displayed in

Fig. 2, the output of step 2 consists of three components including the web interfaces as well as initial database schema and domain logic design.

3. Following step 2, a review session is conducted among developers and clinicians during which the web interface is demonstrated. Clinicians provide feedback on aspects to improve and achieve agreement with developers. With this feedback, the developers repeat step 2 and hold subsequent review sessions. Although loop between step 2 and 3 can happen several times until no changes are requested, it usually ends after two review sessions. Developers can respond to the feedback from clinicians and reduce unmet requirements.

4. At the end of step 3, web interface, database schema, and domain logic design are completed. In this last step, we create database tables and implement detailed domain logic to support the already-built web interface. The deployed version of the system that clinicians interact with is identical to what is finalized in step 3.

Using the WIDD approach, users participate not only in requirements elicitation (step1) but also in system design (step 3). This minimizes the difference between users' expectations and developers' implementation strategies, which in turn improves productivity.

3.2   Data Organization and Access

Neuro3D organizes data capture interfaces according to the types of clinical visit as shown in Fig. 3. The data entry flow in Neuro3D mirrors the clinical workflow to ensure efficient data capture during patient care. A clinical visit consists of a visit date, multiple visit providers, a visit type as "Neurologist Visit," "Neurosurgeon Visit," or "Neuropsychologist Visit," and multiple components captured in Neuro3D. Since data captured in each clinical visit is timestamped, and any piece of patient data is located in some clinical visit, our data organization strategy supports temporal queries.

Role-Based Data Access. People working in a clinical setting have well-defined roles and each role has its own previleges. Each role has a set of privileges and these privileges enable users to perform specific operations. The most common roles in Neuro3D are attending clinician and clinical staff. Attending clinician can view patient data, enter patient data, and review or edit the data entered by other people while clinical staff cannot edit data entered by others.

Patient Data Query, Display, and Navigation. With a large amount of patient data to be captured in Neuro3D, a mechanism is needed for clinicians to search for patients. If an individual patient's name or Medical Record Number is readily available, performing lookup is straightforward.

However, there are other scenarios where lookup with specific patient information is not sufficient. More frequently used patient queries in a DBS program are questions such as "Who are ready for care conference?" Before the deployment of Neuro3D, there is no simple way to answer such questions. Clinicians had

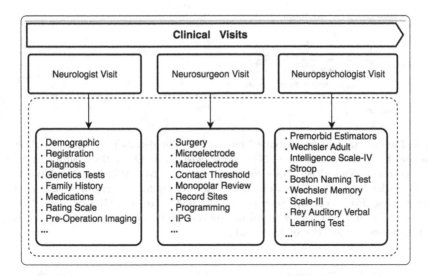

Fig. 3. Data organization by clinical visits in Neuro3D.

to go through all patient records and check if they meet all the pre-conditions for care conference, one by one.

Neuro3D solves this problem by introducing the notion of *patient status*. Patients for DBS intervention go through a number of common clinical procedures as shown in Fig. 1. Neuro3D defines 13 patient statuses (left of Fig. 4) to represent 13 different stages in the DBS workflow. Each box represents a patient status. The coloring of the status box reflects its possible state: *green* indicates "completed" or "confirmed," *red* means "incomplete" or "negative," and *white* represents "unknown." Status change is automatically triggered during data entry. For example, the **I** status (interested in DBS) of a patient is changed from *white* to *green* once a registration form is entered, in which the field "interested in DBS" in registration form is selected as "Yes."

Neuro3D builds on the technique of patient status described above to create a concise patient search interface. The patient search interface uses the 13 patient status boxes as the template and the configuration of the selected colors for the intended results. One can click to change individual status box to red, green, or white. With patient status information stored in Neuro3D, this patient search interface can find all patients satisfying certain criteria expressed by the query template. For example, to answer the question "Who are ready for care conference," clinicians just need to perform 7 clicks on all status boxes in the template before **C** to make them green, two clicks on **C** to make it red, leaving the status for the rest of the boxes as is (white). The patient search interface returns a list of patients satisfying the conditions specified in the template. Each patient record has its status array displayed in its record row. Each box in the status array provides additional information about the status of the specific patient via mouse-over. As shown on the bottom left of Fig. 4, when mouse hovering over

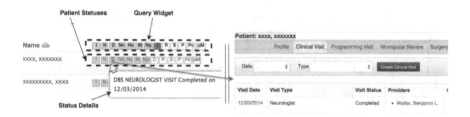

Fig. 4. Patient statuses are displayed on the left. The details of the status abbreviations are: **I** – Interested in DBS, **N** – Neurologist Visit, **D** – DBS Neurologist Visit, **Nn** – Neurology Nurse Visit, **Ns** – Neurosurgery Visit, **M** – MRI Imaging, **Np** – Neuropsychologist Visit, **C** – Care Conference, **R** – Ready for Surgery, **S** – Surgery, **P** – Programming, **Po** – Post-Op Neuropsych, and **pM** – Post-Op MRI Imaging. Mouse-over the status area will trigger the display of the label for explanation of the meaning for each status symbol. (Color figure online)

status box **D**, it shows DBS neurologist visit was completed on 12/03/2014. In addition, a user can click the patient status box to display the relevant data forms. As illustrated in Fig. 4, clicking on the status box **D** leads to clinical visit forms on 12/03/2014 of the patient (right of Fig. 4).

4   Results

Since April 2014, Neuro3D has been deployed in the Movement Disorders Center at the University Hospitals in Cleveland, which is recognized extensively for its treatment of PD. DBS is one of the most innovative and effective techniques used in the center. Neuro3D captured 236 patient records. Clinicians rely on it not only to capture new patient data but also document previous patients who have completed the procedure. Using Neuro3D's patient search interface, we obtain the statistics about the patients captured in the system displayed in Fig. 5 using queries that are most useful in the DBS program. Query 1 and 2 found 23 of 236 who are interested in DBS and 39 who are not interested while the other 174 are undecided. Further inspection of patient data shows that 172 of those 174 patients have already completed the DBS procedure. Patient status usually turns into "not interested" in DBS after the operation is performed. Query 4 indicates that 38 of the 39 patients who are not interested in DBS is because of the completion of their surgeries. Query 11 found patients with care conference completed but are still not ready for surgery. The rest of the queries are frequently used for finding patients that are ready for some clinical procedure or visit such as neurologist visit, care conference, or MRI, but those procedures or visits have not been scheduled. Such query results are easily validated using the direct links to the respective data forms provided in the resulting status arrays.

#	Sample Clinical Query	Status Template	Results
1	All patients in Neuro3D	I N D Nn Ns M Np C R S P Po pM	236
2	Patients that are interested in DBS procedure	I N D Nn Ns M Np C R S P Po pM	23
3	Patients are not interested in DBS procedure	I N D Nn Ns M Np C R S P Po pM	39
4	Patients that have surgery done and become not interested in DBS	I N D Nn Ns M Np C R S P Po pM	38
5	Patients that need be scheduled for neurologist visit	I N D Nn Ns M Np C R S P Po pM	1
6	Patients that need be scheduled for neurology nurse visit	I N D Nn Ns M Np C R S P Po pM	12
7	Patients that need be scheduled for neurosurgery visit	I N D Nn Ns M Np C R S P Po pM	8
8	Patients that need to do MRI Imaging	I N D Nn Ns M Np C R S P Po pM	9
9	Patients that are ready for neuropsychology	I N D Nn Ns M Np C R S P Po pM	6
10	Patients that are ready for care conference	I N D Nn Ns M Np C R S P Po pM	6
11	Patients that have care conference but not ready for surgery	I N D Nn Ns M Np C R S P Po pM	2
12	Patients that are ready to have DBS operation	I N D Nn Ns M Np C R S P Po pM	2
13	Patients have surgery done but programming is not scheduled	I N D Nn Ns M Np C R S P Po pM	0
14	Patients that need post-op neuropsychology	I N D Nn Ns M Np C R S P Po pM	1
15	Patients that need post-op MRI imaging	I N D Nn Ns M Np C R S P Po pM	1

Fig. 5. Statistics about patient statuses captured in Neuro3D

5   Evaluation

Neuro3D consists of 36 forms shown in Fig. 1. These forms contain 1,109 data fields (see Table 2). Each data field captures essential information about PD patients. Following WIDD agile methodology, we created two types of web interfaces for these forms – one for data entry and the other for data display. In total, Neuro3D has more than 72 distinct web pages for patient data capture and display.

In addition to capturing new patient data for DBS, Neuro3D is also used to document historic patients, which demonstrates its generality and effectiveness in the data representation. Figure 6 shows the yearly number of patients recorded in Neuro3D. Patient number has been increasing constantly since the deployment of Neuro3D in 2014. Patient number (32) by August of 2016 is greater than the number (31) of the whole year in 2013.

Table 2. Distinct forms in Neuro3D and the number of data fields captured

Form name	Data fields	Form name	Data fields
Demographic	30	DBS Neuropsychology	127
Registration	19	Post-Op Imaging	13
Diagnosis	15	Care Conference	28
Genetics	10	Procedure Plan	5
DNA Test	5	Surgery	20
Family History	13	Microelectrode	19
Initial Medications	10	Macroelectrode	22
Final Medications	10	Monopolar Review	17
UPDRS	76	Programming	45
MDS–UPDRS	60	Battery and Lead Impedance	32
TRS	56	Therapy Impedance	7
BFMDRS	45	OR Contact Threshold	10
TWSTRS	36	IPG	11
UDRS	47	Record Site	14
Epworth	17	Micro/Macro Stimulation Site	26
MMSE	20	Post-Op Neuropsych	127
MoCA	46	Post-Op Imaging	13
SF36	41	Adverse Event	17

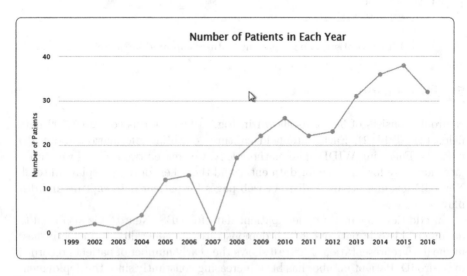

Fig. 6. Patients in Neuro3D by year: 31 in year 2013, 36 in year 2014, 38 in 2015, and 32 in first half of year 2016.

6   Discussion

WIDD is a novel type of agile software development approach. In typical iterative and incremental software development, a function is designed, developed and tested in repeated cycles [15,17]. However, data model schema and business logic are rarely precisely defined at early cycles. This requires developers to frequently revise these implementations in later cycles when the system is better understood which empirically takes great time and efforts. In contrast, WIDD starts with the design and implementation of web interfaces and obtains clients (e.g., clinicians in Neuro3D) close involvement in the iterative revisions of the interfaces until they are satisfied. Meanwhile, data model design and business logic design are also finalized. WIDD successfully defers the implementation of data models and business logic to the last steps before deployment to save developers efforts required to refactor these two modules.

A limitation of the current contribution is the lack of formal user evaluations. In the future, we plan to systematically evaluate: (1) the improvement of WIDD compared to traditional incremental software development; and (2) Neuro3D's positive impact on DBS procedures.

7   Conclusion

Thousands of PD patients undergo DBS surgery each year in an attempt to better control their symptoms and alleviate the burden of the disease. However, universal consensus on best practices for the surgical placement and medical management of DBS systems remains undefined. Neuro3D is well positioned to address such issues and produces direct impact on clinical care. The successful deployment of Neuro3D can bring improvements in three aspects of clinical DBS practice. First, as a clinical database system it can help standardize clinical visits and data collection; Second, capture and management of patient electrode implantation data can help plan the electrode trajectory pre-operatively; Third, capture and management of electrode programming data can assist patient to achieve optimal setting for implanted electrodes; Fourth, Neuro3D's data query and navigation improves clinician's ability to identify patient cohorts efficiently.

In this paper, we present Neuro3D, a flexible and scalable web-based application that actively capture clinical DBS data of PD patients. It allows clinicians to participate in the system design and implementation with Web Interface-Driven Development methodology; it uses core specific role based access control to ensure the correct levels of visibility of data to every user; and it introduces patient status concepts and clinical visit as the portal for patient data to enable efficient data navigation.

Acknowledgement. The work was supported by University of Kentucky Center for Clinical and Translational Science (Clinical and Translational Science Award UL1TR0001998).

References

1. Parkinson's Disease Information Page. NINDS. 21 July 2016. http://www.ninds. nih.gov/disorders/parkinsons_disease/parkinsons_disease.htm. Accessed 2 Aug 2016
2. Statistics on Parkinson's. PDF. http://www.pdf.org/en/parkinson_statistics. Accessed 2 Aug 2016
3. Dorsey, E., Constantinescu, R., Thompson, J., Biglan, K., Holloway, R., Kieburtz, K., Marshall, F., Ravina, B., Schifitto, G., Siderowf, A., Tanner, C.: Projected number of people with Parkinson disease in the most populous nations, 2005 through 2030. Neurology **68**(5), 384–386 (2007)
4. Drew, S.K., Rajeev, K.: Deep brain stimulation. Neurologist **13**, 237–252 (2007)
5. Sorin, B., Jorg, B.S., Alim-Louis, B.: Deep brain stimulation. Cell Tissue Res. **318**, 275–288 (2004)
6. Rubino, J.T.: Interpersonal psychotherapy for depression in Parkinson's disease (Doctoral dissertation, Rutgers University-Graduate School of Applied and Professional Psychology) (2013)
7. Rascol, O., Brooks, D., Korczyn, A., De, P., Clarke, C., Lang, A.: A five-year study of the incidence of dyskinesia in patients with early Parkinson's disease who were treated with ropinirole or levodopa. N. Engl. J. Med. **342**, 1484–1491 (2000)
8. Raja, M., Eugene, L.: Deep brain stimulation in Parkinson's disease. Transl. Neurodegeneration **2**, 22 (2013)
9. Gabbard, G.: Mind, brain, and personality disorders. Am. J. Psychiatry **162**, 648–655 (2005)
10. Shaheen, L., Enoch, C.: Deep brain stimulation for obsessive-compulsive disorder and treatment-resistant depression: systematic review. BMC Res. Notes **3**, 60 (2010)
11. Malone, D., Dougherty, D., Rezai, A., Carpenter, L., Friehs, G., Eskandar, E., et al.: Deep brain stimulation of the ventral capsule/ventral striatum for treatment-resistant depression. Biol. Psychiatry. **65**(4), 267–275 (2009)
12. Ravi, S., Edward, C., Hal, F., Charles, Y.: Role-based access control models. IEEE Comput. **29**(2), 38–47 (1996)
13. Lee, A., Lochovsky, F.H.: User interface design. In: Tsichritzis, D.C. (ed.) Office Automation. Topics in Information Systems, pp. 3–20. Springer, Heidelberg (1985)
14. Deborah, M.: Principles and Guidelines in Software User Interface Design. Prentice-Hall Inc., Upper Saddle River (1991)
15. Martin, C.: Agile Software Development: Principles, Patterns, and Practices. Prentice Hall PTR, Upper Saddle River (2003)
16. Christopher, G., Barbara, T., et al.: Movement disorder society-sponsored revision of the unified Parkinson's disease rating scale (MDS-UPDRS): scale presentation and clinimetric testing results. Mov. Dis. **23**, 2129–2170 (2008)
17. Larman, C., Victor, B.: Iterative and incremental development: a brief history. Computer **36**(6), 47–56 (2003)

A Novel Algorithm to Determine the Cutoff Score

Xiaodong Wang[2], Jun Tian[3], and Daxin Zhu[1(✉)]

[1] Quanzhou Normal University, Quanzhou 362000, China
dex@qztc.edu.cn
[2] Fujian University of Technology, Fuzhou 350108, China
[3] Fujian Medical University, Fuzhou 350004, China

Abstract. The measuring resilience of the patients with cancer can help the clinic doctors and nurses screen the patients with poor resilience, so that they can provide the patients psychological care and intervention in time. In this paper, the ROC curve combining with polynomial regression are used to determine the cutoff score, and the program of analysis is described.

1 Introduction

Cancer is a kind of disease of serious harm to human health. Once they are diagnosed with cancer, patients are often under great emotional and psychological blow [1]. The patient's quality of life has been greatly affected after they undergo surgery and chemoradiation [2–4]. However, many studies have found that in patients with the same disease and cancer treatment situations, their quality of life can make a big difference [5,6]. Psychologists believe that psychological resilience is the main reason for the patients with the same condition having a different feel on their quality of life [7,8]. Psychological resilience is the ability for individuals to regulate them returning to normal when they face unfortunate events [8]. Cancer patients with good mental flexibility are able to regulate their positive attitude to deal with the disease and treatment in a shorter time. Therefore, the measurement of psychological resilience of cancer patients enables clinicians and nurses to determine the patients need to be focused on psychological care and intervention.

RS-14 is now a flexible tool used worldwide to measure the psychological resilience [9]. The scale has 14 entries. Each entry is rated from 1 (strongly disagree) to 7 (completely agree). The tested people scored himself, according to his own situation between 1–7. Scale scores up to 98 points, the lowest was 14 points. The higher the scale score, the better the resilience. A positive diagnosis of community values must be determined when RS-14 is used to screen for the clinic patients with weak psychological resilience. For a diagnostic index, the diagnostic cutoff value is usually determined by the Youden index method [10]. For quantitative indices of continuous values, the diagnostic cutoff values determined by the method are not precise enough.

X. Yin et al. (Eds.): HIS 2016, LNCS 10038, pp. 43–48, 2016.
DOI: 10.1007/978-3-319-48335-1_5

ROC curve is referred to as the receiver operating characteristic curve. In medical decision-making, ROC curves are commonly used to evaluate the results of diagnostic test [11]. The curve parameters can be estimated by drawing a ROC curve according to the index measurement data of index positive and negative of the observed objects. This paper will use the ROC curve to determine the reference cutoff value for low resilience of the clinical cancer patients in RS-14. Our findings can provide useful information for clinical doctors and nurses to screen and find out the patients with weak resilience, so as to give them psychological care and intervention timely.

2   The Description of Our Methods

2.1   Drawing a ROC Curve

Step 1: Grouping the patients.
Patients with severe symptoms of anxiety or severe depressive symptoms were divided into a group (true positive group). Patients with neither serious anxiety nor severe depressive symptoms were divided into another group (true negative).

Step 2: Calculating the cutoff points.
We first calculate the extreme difference of resilience scores in all patients. Then we set the group distance to be the calculated extreme difference divided by 10. The first cutoff point must be the minimum of the resilience scores plus the group distance. The second cutoff point is then the first cutoff point plus the group distance, and so on. We obtain a total of 10 cutoff points.

Step 3: Drawing the curve.
We first calculate the sensitivities S_e (true positive rate) and the specificities S_p (true negative rate) for each cutoff point respectively. Then we build a coordinate system with $1 - S_p$ as its horizontal axis and S_e as its vertical axis. In this coordinate system, we plot the points and connect them into a curve. This is the ROC curve we want.

2.2   The Area Under the ROC Curve

The size of the area under the ROC curve reflects the diagnostic capabilities of diagnostic indices. If a diagnostic index has a good ability of diagnosis, then the sensitivity and specificity with the changing of diagnostic cutoff values will have the following features: The specificity $S_p = 1$ ($1 - S_p = 0$), when $S_e = 0$; The specificity $S_p = 0$ ($1 - S_p = 1$), when $S_e = 1$; The values of S_p will decrease slowly ($1 - S_p$ increase slowly), when the values of S_e increase rapidly. The ROC curves have these variation characteristics will have a shape like a rectangle. So in this case, the area under the ROC curve is approximately the area of a rectangle, which equals the length of the rectangle multiplies the width of the rectangle, i.e. $1 \times 1 = 1$.

If a diagnostic index does not have an ability of diagnosis, then for each of diagnosed person, according to the index the diagnosis with a positive result and a negative result will have the same probability 50 %. Thus, for all the sensitivities and specificities calculated from possible diagnostic cutoff values, we have, $S_e = 1 - S_p$. In this case, the ROC curve becomes a straight line $S_e = 1 - S_p$. So the area under the ROC curve is a half of the area of a rectangle. That is 0.5.

Therefore, the closer to 1 the area under the ROC curve, the stronger the diagnostic capability of the index; the closer to 0.5 the area under the ROC curve, the weaker the diagnostic capability of the index.

We can calculate the area under the ROC curve by the following method. Let the diagnostic index be normally distributed as $N(\mu_0, \sigma_0^2)$ in the population of non-patients. The sample size of patients is n_1, and the sample size of non-patients is n_0.

If $\mu_1 > \mu_0$, then set $\hat{a} = \frac{(\hat{\mu}_1 - \hat{\mu}_0)}{\hat{\sigma}_1}$, $\hat{b} = \frac{\hat{\sigma}_0}{\hat{\sigma}_1}$.

If $\mu_1 < \mu_0$, then set $\hat{a} = \frac{(\hat{\mu}_0 - \hat{\mu}_1)}{\hat{\sigma}_1}$, $\hat{b} = \frac{\hat{\sigma}_0}{\hat{\sigma}_1}$.

Where $\hat{\mu}_0, \hat{\sigma}_0, \hat{\mu}_1, \hat{\sigma}_1$ are the sample estimation of $\mu_0, \sigma_0, \mu_1, \sigma_1$ respectively. The area under the ROC curve is then:

$$\hat{A} = \Phi\left(\frac{\hat{a}}{\sqrt{1 + \hat{b}^2}}\right) \tag{1}$$

where $\Phi(u)$ is the area under the standard normal distribution curve in the range $(-\infty, u)$.

The estimated variance of $\hat{A}$ in formula (1) is

$$Var(\hat{A}) = f^2 Var(\hat{a}) + g^2 Var(\hat{b}) + 2fg Cov(\hat{a}, \hat{b}) \tag{2}$$

2.3 Determine the Diagnostic Cutoff Values

We can determine the diagnostic cutoff values in the following 5 steps.

Step 1: Determine the effective value of decision.

The effective value $C_{TP} = 1.0$ if patients were diagnosed correctly and effective treatments were provided. The effective value $C_{TN} = 0.9$ if non-patients were diagnosed correctly and no treatments were provided. The effective value $C_{FP} = 0.7$ if non-patients were misdiagnosed and unnecessary treatments were provided. The effective value $C_{FN} = 0.0$ if patients were misdiagnosed and no effective treatments were provided.

Step 2: Calculate the slope of the optimal point of the ROC curve.

The slope η of the optimal point of the ROC curve can be calculated by

$$\eta = \frac{(C_{FP} - C_{TN})}{(C_{FN} - C_{TP})} \times \frac{1 - p}{p} \tag{3}$$

where p is the incidence of the disease to be diagnosed in the population.

Step 3: Calculate S_e^* and $FPR^* = 1 - S_p^*$ for the optimal point.

If $\hat{b} = 1$ then

$$\begin{cases} S_e^* = \Phi\left(\frac{1}{2} - \frac{\ln \eta}{\hat{a}}\right) \\ FPR^* = \Phi\left(-\frac{\hat{a}}{2} - \frac{\ln \eta}{\hat{a}}\right) \end{cases} \tag{4}$$

If $\hat{b} \neq 1$ then

$$
\begin{cases}
S_e^* = \Phi\left(\dfrac{\hat{a}-\hat{b}\sqrt{\hat{a}^2+(1-\hat{b}^2)\ln\frac{\eta}{b}}}{1-\hat{b}^2}\right) \\[3mm]
FPR^* = \Phi\left(\dfrac{\hat{a}\hat{b}-\sqrt{\hat{a}^2+2(1-\hat{b}^2)\ln\frac{\eta}{b}}}{1-\hat{b}^2}\right)
\end{cases}
\tag{5}
$$

Step 4: Fit the polynomial equation.

Let Z_{S_e} be the Z value while S_e is the right area of the standard normal distribution.

For all possible cutoff values c_i of the index, compute the corresponding sensitivities S_i^e, and then compute Z_{S^i} for all $1 \leq i \leq k$.

With these values we can build a polynomial equation to fit the points $(c_i, Z_{S_e^i})$ for all $1 \leq i \leq k$ as follows.

$$
c = b_0 + b_1 Z_{S_e} + b_2 Z_{S_e}^2
\tag{6}
$$

Step 5: Calculate the sensitivity and specificity.

Substitute S_e^* into the polynomial equation (6) to calculate the corresponding value of c. This value is exactly the optimal diagnostic cutoff value of the diagnostic index. The sensitivity and specificity corresponding to the diagnostic cutoff value are S_e^* and S_p^* respectively.

3   Concluding Remarks

In the process of cancer treatment, side effects arising from treatment often lead to serious psychological problems in the patients with poor resilience. If we can measure their resilience of the cancer patients before starting their treatment, and pay more attention to their psychological care and psychological intervention for the patients with weak resilience in the next course of their treatment, then we can reduce the psychological problems of the patients, thereby reduce the side effects of treatment of patients and improving their quality of life.

In order to find the patients with weak resilience by using RS-14, we have to determine a cutoff value of RS-14 scores of weak psychological resilience. In this research, we have introduced the ROC curve method to determine the cutoff value of RS-14 scores. Compared with the Youden method which typically determine the cutoff value of the maximum Youden index of RS-14 scores, our new method considers the overall rate of weak resilience and the effectiveness of the method under various circumstances, and therefore has better sensitivity. Meanwhile, in the case of the continuous quantitative variables, the cutoff value determined by our method is more reasonable.

In the process of calculating the slope of the ROC curve, we have assumed that the rate of the weak resilience of tumor patients is about 60 %. This assumption is based on the reported incidence of psychological problems in cancer patients is about 54 % [12]. Since the occurrence of psychological problems and the weak resilience are closely related, so we use the incidence of psychological problems as an estimation of the rate of weak resilience. It is obvious that the different P values will result in different cutoff values determined by our method. Therefore, a good background knowledge of the problem should be studied in advance in the application of this method.

A total of 10 cutoff points have been selected in fitting the ROC curve in this paper. If some more cutoff points are selected, the fitting residuals of the polynomial curve will be smaller, and thus the calculated c value will have a smaller estimation error. In practice, we can generate sufficient number of cutoff points by software packages.

In this research, we have also calculated the optimal cutoff points of RS-14 by using the traditional Youden index method. The results showed that the cutoff value of RS-14 determined by the traditional Youden index method is much larger than that of the ROC curve and hence have a low sensitivity of the screening. If this method is used in clinical misdiagnosis, then it may result in a higher misdiagnosis rate. Therefor, we believe that the ROC curve method is a good method to determine the optimal diagnostic cutoff value, and it is worthy of widespread use.

Acknowledgement. This work was supported by Fujian Provincial Key Laboratory of Data-Intensive Computing and Fujian University Laboratory of Intelligent Computing and Information Processing.

References

1. Bottomley, A.: The cancer patient and quality of life. Oncologist **7**, 120–125 (2002)
2. Efficace, F., Bottomley, A., van Andel, G.: Health related quality of life in prostate carcinoma patients: a systematic review of randomized controlled trials. Cancer **97**, 377–388 (2003)
3. Andersen, B.L.: Quality of life for women with gynecologic cancer. Curr. Opin. Obstet. Gynecol. **7**, 69–76 (1995)
4. Arora, N.K., Gustafson, D.H., Hawkins, R.P., McTavish, F., Cella, D.F., Pingree, S., Mendenhall, J.H., Mahvi, D.M.: Impact of surgery and chemotherapy on the quality of life of younger women with breast carcinoma: a prospective study. Cancer **92**, 1288–1298 (2001)
5. Joanne, L., Christine, E.: Exploring links between the concepts of quality of life and resilience. Pediatr. Rehabil. **4**(4), 209–216 (2001)
6. Epping-Jordan, J.E., Compas, B.E., Osowiecki, D.M., et al.: Psychological adjustment in breast cancer processes of emotional distress. Health Psychol. **18**(4), 315–326 (1999)
7. Yi, J.P., Vitaliano, P.P., Smith, R.E., et al.: The role of resilience on psychological adjustment and physical health in patients with diabetes. Br. J. Health Psychol. **13**, 311–325 (2008)
8. Richardson, G.E.: The metatheory of resilience and resiliency. J. Clin. Psychol. **58**, 307–321 (2002)
9. Wagnild, G.M., Young, H.M.: Development and psychometric evaluation of the Resilience Scale. J. Nurs. Meas. **1**(2), 165–178 (1993)

10. Grmec, S., Gasparovic, V.: Comparison of APACHE II, MEES and Glasgow Coma Scale in patients with nontraumatic coma for prediction of mortality. Crit. Care **5**, 19–23 (2001)
11. Hilden, J.: The area under the ROC curve and its competitors. Med. Decis. Making **11**, 95–101 (1991)
12. Tagay, S., Herpertz, S., Langkafel, M., et al.: Health-related quality of life, depression and anxiety in thyroid cancer patients. Care Rehabil. **15**(4), 695–703 (2006)

Knowledge Services Using Rule-Based Formalization for Eligibility Criteria of Clinical Trials

Zhisheng Huang[1(✉)], Qing Hu[1,3], Annette ten Teije[1], Frank van Harmelen[1], and Salah Ait-Mokhtar[2]

[1] Department of Computer Science, VU University Amsterdam,
Amsterdam, The Netherlands
{huang,qhu400,annette,Frank.van.Harmelen}@cs.vu.nl
[2] Xerox Research Centre Europe, Meylan, France
salah.ait-mokhtar@xrce.xerox.com
[3] College of Computer Science and Technology,
Wuhan Univesity of Science and Technology, Wuhan, China

Abstract. Rule-based formalization of eligibility criteria in clinical trials have distinguished features such as declaration, easy maintenance, reusability, and expressiveness. In this paper, we present several knowledge services which can be provided by the rule-based formalization of eligibility criteria. The rule-based formalization can be generated automatically by using the logic programming Prolog with the support of NLP tools for the semantic annotation and relation extraction with medical ontologies/terminologies such as UMLS and SNOMED CT. We show how those automatically generated rule-based formalization for eligibility criteria can be used for the patient recruitment service in SemanticCT, a semantically-enabled system for clinical trials.

1 Introduction

The rule-based formalization of eligibility criteria in clinical trials has many distinguished features. It is expected to be efficient and effective to provide knowledge services in medical applications, because of the following features [7,8].

- **Declaration**. A rule-based formalization is a declarative language that expresses the logic of a computation which needs no exactly description of its control flow. That is significantly different from the procedural programming languages, like Java and many others. A declarative approach of formalization is more suitable for knowledge representation and reasoning. Thus, a rule-based formalization of eligibility criteria would provide a more convenient way for the automatic patient recruitment in clinical trials, compared with other procedural approaches, like script-based formalization, and pattern-based approaches, like SPARQL querying [7].
- **Easy Maintenance**. A rule-based formalization provides an approach in which specified knowledge is easy to be understood for human users, because

© Springer International Publishing AG 2016
X. Yin et al. (Eds.): HIS 2016, LNCS 10038, pp. 49–61, 2016.
DOI: 10.1007/978-3-319-48335-1_6

they are very close to human knowledge. It would not be too hard for human users to check the correctness of the specification of eligibility criteria if they are formalized as a set of rules. Furthermore, changing or revising a single rule would not make an effect on other part of the formalization significantly, because the meaning of the specification is usually represented in a specific rule (or a set of specific rules).

- **Reusability**. In a rule-based formalization, a single rule (or a set of rules) is usually considered to be independent from other part of knowledge. It is much more convenient to re-use some rules of a specification of eligibility criteria of a clinical trial in the specification of another clinical trial, compared with those formalizations which use SPARQL queries with regular expressions. Furthermore, some rules which specify common knowledge, like those rules for temporal reasoning, and domain knowledge, like those involved in knowledge of targeted disease, can be designed to be a common library, which can be re-used for the specification of other trials.

- **Expressiveness**. Automatic patient recruitment usually involves comprehensive scenarios of deliberation and decision-making procedures. It usually requires a sophisticated data processing in workflows. An expressive rule-based language can support various functionalities of workflow processing.

In this paper, we will present several knowledge services which can be provided by the rule-based formalization of eligibility criteria. The rule-based formalization can be generated automatically by using the logic programming Prolog with the support of NLP tools for the semantic annotation and relation extraction with well-known medical ontologies/terminologies such as UMLS and SNOMED CT. In particular, we will show those automatically generated rule-based formalization of eligibility criteria can be used for the patient recruitment service in SemanticCT, a semantically-enabled system for clinical trials [8].

The rest of this paper is organized as follows: Sect. 2 describes the basic idea of rule-based formalization for clinical trials, and discusses the knowledge services which can be provided by them. Section 3 discusses how we can use the Xerox NLP for the natural language text processing in eligibility criteria and how the rule-based formalization can be generated automatically by using the logic programming language Prolog. Section 4 presents how those automatically generated rule-based formalization can be used for the patient recruitment service for clinical trials. Section 5 discusses future work and make the conclusions.

2 Rule-Based Formalization for Clinical Trials

2.1 Eligibility Criteria

Eligibility criteria consist of inclusion criteria, which state a set of conditions that must be met, and exclusion criteria, which state a set of conditions that must not be met, in order to participate in a clinical trial.

Example 1: The eligibility criteria of Trial NCT00002720.

```
DISEASE CHARACTERISTICS:
  - Histologically proven stage I, invasive breast cancer
  - Hormone receptor status:
    - Estrogen receptor positive
    - Progesterone receptor positive or negative
PATIENT CHARACTERISTICS:
  Age: 65 to 80, Sex: Female, Menopausal status: Postmenopausal
  Other: - No serious disease that would preclude surgery
         - No other prior or concurrent malignancy except basal cell
           carcinoma or carcinoma in situ of the cervix
```

In this example, the inclusion criteria and the exclusion criteria are stated explicitly without the heading of the inclusion criteria and the exclusion criteria. For example, 'invasive breast cancer' is an inclusion criterion, and "No serious disease that would preclude surgery" is an exclusion criterion which can be identified by the negative words such as "No".

2.2 Rule-Based Formalization

In [7], we present an implementation of the rule-based formalization on eligibility criteria for patient recruitment and trial feasibility. The rule-based formalization is developed based on the logic programming language Prolog [16,17]. We formalize the knowledge rules of the specification of eligibility criteria of clinical trials with respect to the following different levels of knowledge: trial-specific knowledge, domain-specific knowledge, and common knowledge.

- **Trial-specific Knowledge.** Trial-specific knowledge is those rules which specify the concrete details of the eligibility criteria of a specific clinical trial. Those criteria are different from a trial to another trial. In order to check if a patient meets an inclusion criterion, we can check if its patient data meet the criterion. We introduce a special predicate getNotYetCheckedItems to collect those criteria which have not yet been formalized for the trial.

Here is an example of the formalized inclusion criteria in the trial NCT00002720:

```
meetInclusionCriteria(_PatientID, PatientData, CT, NotYetCheckedItems):-
                CT = 'nct00002720',
                breast_cancer_stage(PatientData, '1'),
                invasive_breast_cancer(PatientData),
                er_positive(PatientData),
                known_pr_status(PatientData),
                age_between(PatientData, 65, 80),
                postmenopausal(PatientData),
                getNotYetCheckedItems(CT, NotYetCheckedItems).
```

Which states that the inclusion criteria include: (i) Histologically proven stage I, invasive breast cancer, (ii) Hormone receptor status: Estrogen receptor positive and Progesterone receptor positive or negative, (iii) Age: 65 to 80, and (iv) Menopausal status: Postmenopausal.

- **Domain-specific Knowledge**. Those trial-specific rules above may involve some knowledge which are domain relevant, i.e., the domain knowledge, which are trial independent. We formalize those part of knowledge in the libraries of domain-specific knowledge. For example, for clinical trials of breast cancer, we formalize the knowledge of breast cancer in the knowledge bases of breast cancer, a domain-specific library of rules. An example of this type of knowledge is a patient of breast cancer is triple negative if the patient has estrogon receptor negative, progesterone receptor negative and protein HER2 negative status. It can be formalized in Prolog as follows:

```
triple_negative(Patient):- er_negative(Patient),
                           pr_negative(Patient),
                           her2_negative(Patient).
```

- **Common Knowledge**. The specification of the eligibility criteria may involve some knowledge which are domain independent, like those knowledge for temporal reasoning and the knowledge for manipulating semantic data and interacting with data servers, e.g. how to obtain the data from SPARQL endpoints. We formalize those knowledge in several rule libraries, which can be reusable for different applications.

Here is an example of this type of knowledge is temporal reasoning with constructs like last-month.

```
lastmonth(LastMonth):- today(Today),
   Today = date(_Year, ThisMonth, _Date),
                              ThisMonth > 1,
   LastMonth  is ThisMonth - 1.

lastmonth(LastMonth):- today(Today),
   Today = date(_Year, ThisMonth, _Date),
                              ThisMonth is 1,
                              LastMonth  is 12.
```

2.3   Knowledge Services Using Formalization for Eligibility Criteria of Clinical Trials

There are various knowledge services which can be provided by the rule-based formalization for clinical trials, which can range from the patient recruitment in which finding eligible patients for a trial, into the trial feasibility estimation when a trial is designed. The following are some typical use cases of the rule-based formalization of eligibility criteria:

- **Patient Recruitment**. Given a clinical trial, finding eligible patients for the trial. The formalization of the eligibility criteria would allow computers to check eligibility criteria automatically or semi-automatically with the patient data and match the patient data with eligibility criteria [5,8].

- **Trial Finding/Selection**. Given a patient, more exactly a patient data, finding suitable trials for the patient. In order to enable the procedure for automatic finding, we have to convert textual description of eligibility criteria into a formalized one. In this use case, we have to formalize all of the trials for which the patient should consider to avoid missing trials. Thus, it usually requires the formalizations for over a few hundred, even a few thousands of clinical trials. We know that manual generation of the formalization of eligibility criteria for a single clinical trial is already time consuming. It would make the manual generation of formalization for over a few thousands of clinical trials to be an impossible mission. That justifies the reason why we need automatic generation of the formalization of eligibility criteria [8].
- **Trial Feasibility**. The trial feasibility checking is done at the design time of a clinical trial. Usually we need some templates of clinical trials, so that the design of a clinical trial can be revised from some existing clinical trials. Moreover, in order to make the trial feasibility checking automatically, again we also need the formalization of eligibility criteria [9].
- **Trial Comparison and Similarity**. We usually want to compare different clinical trials for analysis. That can be achieved by a similarity measure among different clinical trials. The formalization of eligibility criteria would be very helpful for us to make such a comparison.
- **Trial Ranking**. Trial ranking would help us to find those most relevant ones for selection or other use cases. Again, the formalization of eligibility criteria would be very useful for us to achieve the trial ranking automatically.

3 Automatic Generation of Rule-Based Formalization for Eligibility Criteria of Clinical Trials

3.1 NLP Tools for Processing Eligibility Criteria

We use the Xerox's NLP tool XMedlan to make the concept identification with well-known medical terminologies such as UMLS and SNOMED CT [1]. We also use the XMedlan to make the relation extraction over textual eligibility criteria and generate their semantic representation of the concept annotation and the extracted relations [3]. We have decided to use XMedLan rather than similar terminology-based concept identifiers, like the MetaMap system [4] or BioPortal text annotator[1], because it is easier to adapt. It can be customized using a single command line with any subset from UMLS-integrated terminologies and even with in-house, non-standard terminologies [2]. Furthermore, although XMedLan and MetaMap seem to have comparable concept identification capabilities on the ShARe/CLEF-2013 corpus (see [11]), we have never had any computational efficiency issues with XMedLan, while MetaMap can have such issues [4,13].

In the beginning, XMedlan make a preprocessing over textual eligibility criteria for a linguistic analysis [1,3]. In this linguistic analysis, the text is tokenized into a sequence of tokens, each token is looked up in a lexicon and assigned all

---

[1] https://bioportal.bioontology.org/annotator.

its possible morpho-syntactic categories and features, and possibly additional semantic features. Sub-sequences of tokens and concept mentions are grouped into syntactic constituents, called chunks, by the parser. Tokens and concepts mentions are linked with syntactic dependency relations. The linguistic parser performs a local and partial semantic analysis of the input sentence and produces semantic annotations.

The concept identifier spots occurrences of medical concepts and entities by identifying, in the input text, exact matches or variants of terms listed in specified terminologies. For each identified concept, it provides the UMLS concept unique identifier (CUI) and terminology-specific codes such as the concepts in SNOMED CT. It also provides the semantic types assigned to the concept in the UMLS semantic network, i.e. general semantic classes.

The annotations produced by the linguistic analyser and the concept identifier are exploited by the relation extraction engine to identify relations and attributes of concepts and entities in the input text. These relations and attributes are expressed as triples, i.e. typed binary relations in the form $\langle Subject, Property, Object \rangle$, and can be serialized in the RDF NTriple format.

Here is an example of the RDF NTriple format of the semantic representation after the NLP tool processing.

```
sctid:e15 ctec:hasTerm "hormonal therapy".
sctid:e15 ctec:hasCUI "C0279025".
sctid:e15 ctec:hasCardinality sctid:e26.
sctid:e26 ctec:hasQuant "no".
sctid:e22 ctec:hasQuant "10".
sctid:e23 ctec:hasQuant "three".
sctid:e27 ctec:hasQuant "35".
sctid:e28 ctec:hasQuant "1.66 percent".
sctid:e29 ctec:isA sct:diagnosis.
sctid:e29 ctec:hasObject sctid:e4.
sctid:e36 ctec:hasText  "Women over the age of 35 with a 5-year predicted
breast cancer risk of at least 1.66 percent or a history of lobular breast
carcinoma in situ, life expectancy of 10 years or more, breast examination
and mammogram without evidence of cancer, no hormonal therapy within three
months prior to randomization, and no history of deep venous thrombosis or
 pulmonary embolism.".
```

We load those semantic representation of eligibility criteria into a triple store which can serve as a SPARQL endpoint for semantic queries. Here is an example of the semantic query to find the age with the exact age value (i.e. a number) and the textual description in the eligibility criteria.

```
select distinct ?trial ?text ?n
where {
?e1 sct:NCTID ?trial.
?e2 ctec:hasCUI "C0001779|C1114365".
?e1 ctec:hasFragment ?e2.
?e1 ctec:hasText ?text.
?e3 ctec:hasQuant ?n.
?e2 ?p ?e3.
}
ORDER BY ?trial
```

3.2   Property Detection for Automatic Generation of Rule-Based Formalization

We use Prolog as the tool to formalize the knowledge for processing eligibility criteria of clinical trials. More exactly we use the DCG (Definite Clause Grammars) rules in Prolog to extract the information in the textual description of eligibility criteria with the help of the semantic analysis and annotation of eligibility criteria.

DCG rules are convenient to express patterns in a natural language text. In DCG rules, those patterns are described as Prolog lists. A DCG is defined by DCG rules. A DCG rule has the form:

```
head --> body.
```

The main advantage of using DCG rules is that we can make partial text checking to obtain the required information from text without fully analysis over all text in the description.

For example, in order to extract the "stage" information of eligibility criteria, we can check whether or not it contains the text which states a stage and ignore other texts. That may lead to the problem that extracted relations are not complete. One of the examples is that it may ignore the negative information about the stage description. That problem can be avoided by the negation checking and processing on certain atomic properties.

We formalize the identification knowledge in a set of Prolog rules, which consist of a set of rule knowledge on atomic property checking. So far we have built a set of rule knowledge which can deal with many basic properties in eligibility criteria such as gender, stage, age, diagnosis, tumor size, etc. The DCG rules in Prolog can provide much richer repositories for the pattern matching over regular expressions, because it is quite easy for Prolog rules to enhance with a domain knowledge for the processing.

Here is the example of (partial) rule knowledge which can identify the "TNM stage" of eligibility criteria, which covers different patterns of stage description.

```
%Patients with Stage II disease
stageText(stage(N)) --> human,
                        with,
                        stage,
                        stagenumber(N),
                        disease.


%Patients with Stage II disease or Stage III
stageText(stage(N2)) --> human,
                         with,
                         stage,
                         stagenumber(_N1),
                         disease,
                         or,
```

```
                          stage,
                          stagenumber(N2).
```

. . . .

We have built rule knowledge which can deal with 13 atomic properties, which include the properties Gender, Age, TNM stage, Diagnosis, Menopausal Status, Tumor size, Lymph Nodes, Pregnancy, Nursing, etc. The rule knowledge for more properties are under development. We use the rule knowledge to obtain the rule-based formalizations for 4664 clinical trials of breast cancer, which have been collected in the website of clinicaltrials.gov. We download those XML data of clinical trails from the website clinicaltrials.gov, and extract the textual descriptions of eligibility criteria from the XML data. The Xerox NLP tool MedLan is used to make the semantic annotations and relation extractions with the medical ontologies SNOMED CT [14] and UMLS and convert those data into RDF NTriple data. Those semantic data are loaded into the triple store LarKC [6,18], so that they can be obtained via the SPARQL endpoints in the LarKC platform.

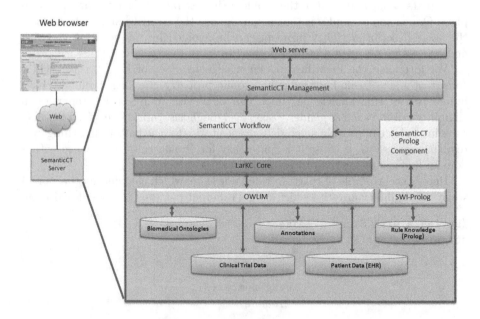

Fig. 1. The architecture of SemanticCT

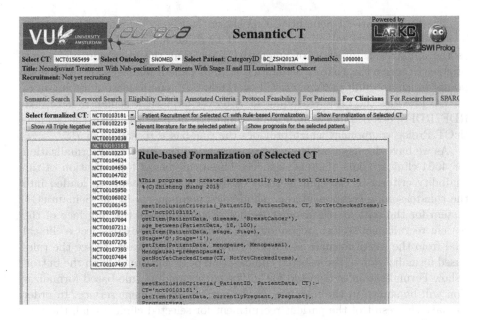

Fig. 2. The interface of SemanticCT

4   Patient Recruitment Service in SemanticCT

SemanticCT is a semantically-enabled system for clinical trials [8][2]. SemanticCT provides the semantic integration of various data in clinical trials. The system is designed to be a semantically enabled system of decision support for various scenarios in medical applications, which include the patient recruitment service, trial feasibility service, trial finding service, medical guidelien update services, and others.

We have used the knowledge-based patient data generator [10] to synthesize the semantic data of 10,000 patients of breast cancer. Those generated data have been loaded into the SemanticCT for the purpose of tests. In SemanticCT, a rule-based formalization is developed based on the logic programming language Prolog. We select the SWI-Prolog[3] as the basic language for the rule-based formalization of eligibility criteria. SWI-Prolog provides a basic tool for the communication with SPARQL endpoints and other REST based web servers. Furthermore, SWI-Prolog also supports the basic reasoning and storage of semantic data. Thus, the SWI-Prolog has the advantage of the support for semantic data processing. SWI-Prolog provides various libraries for data processing, which includes not only the tools for text processing and database-like storage management, but also workflow processing and distributed/parallel processing.

---

[2] http://wasp.cs.vu.nl/sct.

[3] http://www.swi-prolog.org/.

The architecture of SemanticCT is shown in Fig. 1. SemanticCT Management plays a central role of the system. It launches a web server which serves as the application interface of SemanticCT, so that the users can use a web browser to access the system. SemanticCT Management manages SPARQL endpoints which are built as SemanticCT workflows. A generic reasoning plug-in in LarKC provides the basic reasoning service over large-scale semantic data, like RDF/RDFS/OWL data. SemanticCT Management interacts with the SemanticCT Prolog component which provides the rule-based reasoning [5,7].

As we have discussed above, we have generated the rule-based formalization for 4664 clinical trials of breast cancer. Those rule-based formalization of the eligibility criteria in the clinical trials of breast cancer have been loaded into the rule-reasoning component (i.e., the Prolog component) in the SemanticCT system for the patient recruitment service. Figure 2 shows the interface of the patient recruitment service in SemanticCT. Namely the user can select a clinical trial from the list of formalized clinical trials. If the user wants to see the rule-based formalization of the selected clinical trial, he or she can click on the button "Show Formalization of Selected CT". The corresponding rule-based formalization will be shown in the interface of the patient recruitment service. In order to make the result of the patient recruitment for selected clinical trial, the user can click on the button "Patient Recruitment for Selected CT with Rule-based

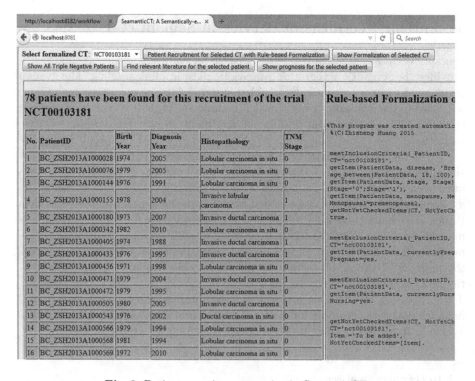

Fig. 3. Patient recruitment service in SemanticCT

Formalization". The result of the patient recruitment will be shown in the left bottom window of the interface as shown in Fig. 3.

5 Discussions and Conclusions

In this paper, we have discussed the main features of rule-based formalization for eligibility criteria of clinical trials. We have presented several knowledge services which can be provided by the rule-based formalization of eligibility criteria for clinical trials. We have proposed to use the DCG rules in the logic programming language Prolog to serve as the formalized knowledge for processing the textual description of eligibility criteria and convert them into the corresponding rule-based formalization of eligibility criteria. We have shown that those automatically generated formalization can provide the patient recruitment service in the SemanticCT system.

In [12], Milian et al. propose an approach of automatic detecting properties from free-text eligibility criteria by defining various patterns with regular expressions in SPARQL queries. Our proposed approach is different from Milian's one, because we define the identification knowledge as a set of rules. As we have discussed in the introduction section, a rule-based formalization provides an approach in which specified knowledge is easy to be understood for human users. Thus, it is much easier for maintenance and reusability. In [15], Tu et al. propose a method for transforming free-text eligibility criteria into computable criteria. The main processing in that method is to fully capture the semantics of criteria directly in a formal expression language by annotating free-text criteria in a format called ERGO annotation. The annotation can be done manually, or it can be partially automated using natural-language processing techniques. Our approach in this paper can provide an automatic generation of the formalizations without manual annotation.

It should be noted that the rule-based formalization is not the only formalization we can use for eligibility criteria of clinical trials. Other formalizations can be developed based on the Semantic Web standards, like RDF/OWL, or on a structured ones, like those based XML data format. As we have discussed before, the rule-based formalization has many distinguished features such as expressiveness and reusability, it is more convenient to accommodate them with the domain knowledge. It should be also noted that Prolog rules are not the only rule-based formalization we can use. There are many other rule-based formalizations such as SWRL rules and description logic rules. Again, as we have discussed before, Prolog rules have the features such as the convenience for the communication with SPARQL endpoints and other REST based web servers.

We are going to implement more knowledge services which can be provided by the rule-based formalization in the SemanticCT as the future work of this paper. The knowledge services in the future work include the trial finding service, the trial comparison and trial similarity measure, and the trial ranking service. Those knowledge services are expected to use in decision support systems for clinical trials.

Acknowledgments. This work is partially supported by the Dutch national project COMMIT/Data2Semantics.

References

1. Ait-Mokhtar, S., Bruijn, B.D., Hagege, C., Rupi, P.: Initial prototype for relation identification between concepts, D3.2. Technical report, EURECA Project (2013)
2. Ait-Mokhtar, S., Bruijn, B.D., Hagege, C., Rupi, P.: Intermediary-stage ie components, D3.5. Technical report, EURECA Project (2014)
3. Aït-Mokhtar, S., Chanod, J.-P., Roux, C.: Robustness beyond shallowness: incremental deep parsing. Nat. Lang. Eng. **8**(2), 121–144 (2002)
4. Aronson, A.R., Lang, F.: An overview of metamap: historical perspective and recent advances. J. Am. Med. Inf. Assoc.: JAMIA **17**(3), 229–236 (2010)
5. Bucur, A., ten Teije, A., van Harmelen, F., Tagni, G., Kondylakis, H., van Leeuwen, J., Schepper, K.D., Huang, Z.: Formalization of eligibility conditions of CT and a patient recruitment method, D6.1. Technical report, EURECA Project (2012)
6. Fensel, D., van Harmelen, F., Andersson, B., Brennan, P., Cunningham, H., Della Valle, E., Fischer, F., Huang, Z., Kiryakov, A., Lee, T., School, L., Tresp, V., Wesner, S., Witbrock, M., Zhong, N.: Towards LarKC: a platform for web-scale reasoning. In: Proceedings of the IEEE International Conference on Semantic Computing (ICSC). IEEE Computer Society Press, CA (2008)
7. Huang, Z., Teije, A., Harmelen, F.: Rule-based formalization of eligibility criteria for clinical trials. In: Peek, N., Marín Morales, R., Peleg, M. (eds.) AIME 2013. LNCS (LNAI), vol. 7885, pp. 38–47. Springer, Heidelberg (2013). doi:10.1007/978-3-642-38326-7_7
8. Huang, Z., ten Teije, A., van Harmelen, F.: SemanticCT: a semantically-enabled system for clinical trials. In: Riaño, D., Lenz, R., Miksch, S., Peleg, M., Reichert, M., ten Teije, A. (eds.) KR4HC/ProHealth -2013. LNCS (LNAI), vol. 8268, pp. 11–25. Springer, Heidelberg (2013). doi:10.1007/978-3-319-03916-9_2
9. Huang, Z., van Harmelen, F., ten Teije, A., Dekker, A.: Feasibility estimation for clinical trials. In: Proceedings of the 7th International Conference on Health Informatics (HEALTHINF 2014), Angers, Loire Valley, France, 3–6 March 2014
10. Huang, Z., van Harmelen, F., ten Teije, A., Dentler, K.: Knowledge-based patient data generation. In: Riaño, D., Lenz, R., Miksch, S., Peleg, M., Reichert, M., ten Teije, A. (eds.) KR4HC/ProHealth 2013. LNCS (LNAI), vol. 8268, pp. 83–96. Springer, Heidelberg (2013). doi:10.1007/978-3-319-03916-9_7
11. Khiari, A.: Identification of variants of compound terms, master thesis. Technical report, Universite Paul Sabatier, Toulouse (2015)
12. Milian, K., Teije, A.: Towards automatic patient eligibility assessment: from free-text criteria to queries. In: Peek, N., Marín Morales, R., Peleg, M. (eds.) AIME 2013. LNCS (LNAI), vol. 7885, pp. 78–83. Springer, Heidelberg (2013). doi:10.1007/978-3-642-38326-7_12
13. Pyysalo, S., Ananiadou, S.: Anatomical entity mention recognition at literature scale. Bioinformatics **30**(6), 868–875 (2014)
14. Spackman, K.: Managing clinical terminology hierarchies using algorithmic calculation of subsumption: Experience with snomed-rt. J. Am. Med. Inf. Assoc. (2000)
15. Tu, S., Peleg, M., Carini, S., Bobak, M., Ross, J., Rubin, D., Sim, I.: A practical method for transforming free-text eligibility criteria into computable criteria. JBI **44**(2), 239–250 (2011)

16. Wielemaker, J., Huang, Z., van der Meij, L.: SWI-Prolog and the web. J. Theory Pract. Logic Program. **8**(3), 363–392 (2008)

17. Wielemaker, J., Schrijvers, T., Triska, M., Lager, T.: SWI-Prolog. J. Theory Pract. Logic Program. **12**(1–2), 67–96 (2012)

18. Witbrock, M., Fortuna, B., Bradesko, L., Kerrigan, M., Bishop, B., van Harmelen, F., ten Teije, A., Oren, E., Momtchev, V., Tenschert, A., Cheptsov, A., Roller, S., Gallizo, G.: D5.3.1 - requirements analysis and report on lessons learned during prototyping. Larkc project deliverable, June 2009

Dietary Management Software for Chronic Kidney Disease: Current Status and Open Issues

Xiaorui Chen[1], Maureen A. Murtaugh[1], Corinna Koebnick[2],
Srinivasan Beddhu[1], Jennifer H. Garvin[1], Mike Conway[1],
Younghee Lee[1], Ramkiran Gouripeddi[1], and Gang Luo[1(✉)]

[1] University of Utah, Salt Lake City, UT 84108, USA
{xiaorui.chen, maureen.murtaugh, srinivasan.beddhu,
jennifer.garvin}@hsc.utah.edu, {mike.conway,
younghee.lee, ram.gouripeddi, gang.luo}@utah.edu
[2] Kaiser Permanente Southern California, Pasadena, CA 91101, USA
Corinna.Koebnick@kp.org

Abstract. Chronic kidney disease (CKD) affects about 10 % of the population worldwide. Millions of people die prematurely from CKD each year. Dietary restrictions can slow the progression of CKD and improve outcomes. In recent years, introduction of new technologies has enabled patients to better manage their own dietary intake and health. Several dietary management software tools are currently available providing personalized nutrition and diet management advice for CKD patients. In this paper, we provide an overview of these software tools and discuss some open issues and possible solutions, in hope of stimulating future research in consumer health informatics for CKD.

Keywords: Chronic kidney disease · Dietary management software · Consumer health informatics

1 Introduction

Chronic kidney disease (CKD) is characterized by a slow, progressive loss of kidney function over a period of time [1]. CKD is defined by abnormalities in kidney function or albuminuria (increased protein in the urine) persisting for at least three months. CKD encompasses a broad range of disease severity and significant heterogeneity in the risk of progression to end-stage renal disease, morbidity, and mortality [2]. Kidney function can be assessed using the estimated glomerular filtration rate (eGFR) computed based on serum creatinine. CKD has five stages, with stage 1 (eGFR $\geq$ 90 mL/min/1.73 m^2) being the mildest and stage 5 (eGFR < 15 mL/min/1.73 m^2) being the most severe [3]. Stage 5 CKD, or end-stage renal disease, requires renal replacement therapy such as dialysis or kidney transplantation to maintain life. Current evidence suggests that a low eGFR increases the risk for complications including anemia, cardiovascular disease, and mineral and bone disease [3].

© Springer International Publishing AG 2016
X. Yin et al. (Eds.): HIS 2016, LNCS 10038, pp. 62–72, 2016.
DOI: 10.1007/978-3-319-48335-1_7

According to Medicare, 10 % of the Medicare population has recognized CKD accounting for more than 20 % of Medicare's total costs in 2013 [4]. Most of these costs were spent on renal replacement therapy. Since CKD is not reversible, interventions can only slow its progression and help prevent complications.

Besides the treatment and control of hypertension, albuminuria, diabetes, and metabolic acidosis, dietary factors play an important role in the progression and outcomes of CKD. A growing body of evidence suggests that precision care provided by a dietitian can help CKD patients maintain their health, slow disease progression, and reduce complications [5]. Although it is expensive to see a dietitian, nutrition therapy provided by the dietitian can delay the need for dialysis or kidney transplant and be cost-effective for patients. However, most CKD patients have an insufficient understanding of their disease and dietary requirements [6]. Few patients receive dietary counseling before developing end-stage renal disease. According to the 2010 United States Renal Data System annual data report, only 3.9 % of CKD patients saw a dietitian for more than one year before starting dialysis [7].

CKD patients have complex dietary needs and ideally should continually monitor their protein, sodium, phosphorus, potassium, and fluid intake. However, patients often have difficulty determining whether food items consumed in unfamiliar environments (e.g., restaurants) conform with their dietitians' recommendations. When shopping for fruits and vegetables in grocery stores, absence of food packaging and nutrition labels can make it difficult for patients to identify their purchases' nutritional content. Further, it is cumbersome for patients to manually track meals, snacks, and drinks consumed throughout the day, calculate their nutrient levels, and compare them to dietitians' recommendations. By helping CKD patients manage their diet, computer-based interventions can fill many of these gaps. In this paper, we discuss the current status and open issues of dietary management software for CKD, with the hope of stimulating future research in consumer health informatics for CKD.

The rest of this paper is organized as follows. Section 2 describes current dietary recommendations for CKD patients. Section 3 shows evidence on existing dietary management software's efficacy for improving diets in the general population. Section 4 gives an overview of existing dietary management software tools for CKD patients. Section 5 presents some open issues and possible solutions. We conclude in Sect. 6.

2 Current Dietary Recommendations for CKD Patients

Kidneys help maintain fluid and electrolyte balance in the body, as well as remove metabolic wastes from the body. A diet appropriate for healthy people can be problematic for CKD patients as their kidney function declines. In CKD patients, over-consumption of certain nutrients can cause hyperkalemia (high blood potassium), hyperphosphatemia (high blood phosphorus), high blood pressure, fluid volume overload, and accumulation of uremic toxins. On the other hand, sarcopenia (muscle loss associated with the aging process) and decreased nutrient intake could contribute to protein-energy wasting [8]. Thus, appropriate nutrition is an important component of CKD management for minimizing complications. A well-balanced diet aims to balance electrolytes, minerals, and fluids in the body and provides appropriate energy to maintain body functions.

Proteins are important building blocks of human body tissues. As kidney function declines, kidneys must work harder to remove waste products from protein metabolism. The Dietary Reference Intakes recommends a daily protein intake of 0.8 g/kg for healthy adults [9]. However, patients with stage 4 CKD are recommended to reduce their daily protein intake to 0.6 g/kg [10] because excessive protein intake can accelerate CKD.

Dietary intake of sodium, phosphorus, and potassium need to be closely monitored and continuously adjusted based on the CKD patient's kidney function, health status, and blood test results. Human body needs sodium, phosphorus, and potassium to work properly. However, as kidneys lose their function, these minerals' intake needs to be limited as kidneys can no longer remove excess minerals from the blood. Excessive sodium intake can elevate blood pressure and body fluid level leading to heart failure. High blood phosphorus level can increase risk of weakened bones and heart disease. Also, high blood potassium level can cause serious consequences such as sudden cardiac death due to arrhythmias.

Some CKD patients such as those on dialysis need to restrict their fluid intake, as their kidneys can no longer remove excess water from the blood. Excessive fluid retention in the circulatory system, body tissues, or cavities in the body cause high blood pressure, edema, and breathing difficulties.

3   Dietary Management Software for the General Population

Computer software holds great promise for delivering personalized nutrition interventions. Research has shown that personalized nutrition education tailored by computers based on survey results obtained from patients can be more effective at motivating patients to make dietary changes than providing general dietary guidelines [11]. Compared to general dietary guidelines, personalized dietary recommendations generated by computers contain less extraneous information and are cognitively processed more intensively, leading to more self-motivating cognitions.

At present, several dietary management software tools are available for weight control in the general population. By simulating face-to-face nutrition counseling and providing personalized nutrition interventions, these software tools help users monitor their eating behavior in a cost-effective way.

Carter et al. developed My Meal Mate, a mobile app tracking users' diet to help lose weight. The app allows users to set a weight loss goal and provides daily calorie allowance for achieving this goal. Users can use the app to log their food intake and physical activities and track their progress. Carter et al. compared the dietary data captured by the app with a duplicate 24-h dietary recall, a gold standard for dietary assessment [12]. The results showed a moderate to strong correlation between the two measurements for calories and macronutrients (i.e., proteins, carbohydrates, and fats) [13]. In a related pilot study conducted on overweight adults, using the app for six months led to an average weight loss of 4.6 kg [14].

Software for dietitians providing hospital care can result in reduced error while saving time. Skouroliakou et al. developed DIET, a software tool that calculates personalized dietary requirements and produces daily menus for hospitalized patients [15]. Skouroliakou et al. evaluated DIET versus traditional face-to-face interventions given by dietitians for calculating dietary and nutrient intake and menu planning in 135 hospitalized patients. Compared to manual methods, using *DIET* reduced calculation errors from 12 % to 1.5 %, which is clinically significant, and also decreased nutrition calculation and menu planning time by 50 %. Hong *et al*. developed *NutriSonic*, a Web-based system for dietary counseling and menu management [16]. *NutriSonic* analyzes meals' nutritional content using computer-generated menus and compares it with Korean Recommended Dietary Allowance. The study showed that *NutriSonic* can not only accurately and quickly calculate users' nutritional needs, but also be used by both dietitians and the general population.

General dietary management software has great potential to improve health for the general population. However, it is not ideally suited for CKD patients for three reasons. First, unlike the general population, CKD patients need to follow a special diet limiting certain nutrients such as proteins, sodium, potassium, phosphorus, and fluids. General dietary management software does not address these special requirements. Second, general dietary management software lacks information of certain nutrient levels in its food database and hence cannot make recommendations based on such information. For instance, *MyFitnessPal*, one of the largest food databases, includes no information on phosphorus level. However, CKD patients need to carefully manage their intake of food with high amounts of phosphorus, such as dairy products, meat, nuts, and beans. Third, dietary recommendations need to be personalized for a CKD patient based on his/her CKD-related health status such as kidney function and comorbidities. General dietary management software does not capture enough health data for this purpose. In summary, general dietary management software does not meet CKD patients' special nutrition demands. CKD patients need customized dietary management software designed and optimized for their need to manage dietary restrictions.

4   An Overview of Existing Dietary Management Software for CKD

Over the past few years, several dietary management software tools specifically designed for CKD patients have been released, including *MyFoodCoach* by the National Kidney Foundation, *Diet Helper* by the company Davita, and *KidneyAPPetite* by the company Sanofi. These software tools have similar functions: creating personalized dietary recommendations and monitoring the user's dietary/nutritional intake. Each of these software tools has one or more of the following components: a health data input interface, a medical knowledge base and inference engine, a diet tracking system, and a diet recommender system.

4.1   Health Data Input Interface

When a user first uses a dietary management software tool for CKD, he/she is required to enter some basic health information about himself/herself. The software tool saves these data in its database and produces personalized dietary recommendations based on these data. Typically requested data elements include demographics (e.g., age, gender, and race), anthropometric measurements (e.g., weight, height, and body mass index), kidney function (e.g., eGFR, whether the patient is on dialysis, and whether the patient has had kidney transplantation), comorbidities and complications (e.g., diabetes and hypertension), and lab test results (e.g., serum potassium levels, serum phosphorus levels, and serum calcium levels).

4.2   Medical Knowledge Base and Inference Engine

A dietary management software tool for CKD usually has a medical knowledge base and an inference engine. The inference engine uses both the medical knowledge stored in the knowledge base and the user's health information stored in the database to produce personalized dietary recommendations. Outputs are in the form of daily allowances for calories, protein, sodium, potassium, phosphorus, water, and other nutrients important for CKD patients.

Medical knowledge is usually stored in the knowledge base in the form of rules. For example, patients with stage 4 CKD ($15 \leq$ eGFR < 30 mL/min/1.73 m^2) are recommended to reduce their daily protein intake to less than 0.6 g/kg. A rule for this can be: if the patient's eGFR is < 30 AND the patient's eGFR is ≥ 15, then the patient's daily allowance for protein $= 0.6 \times$ the patient's weight (kg). As another example, fluid for CKD patients on dialysis is restricted to 1–1.5 L/day. A rule for this can be: if the patient is on dialysis, then the patient's daily allowance for water is 1.5 L.

Although some CKD patients prefer consulting a dietitian or physician for a diet prescription rather than completely relying on computer software, they still need a tool to help them manage their nutritional intake on a daily basis. Some dietary management software tools for CKD give users an option of manually inputting their dietitians' recommendations to override the nutrition allowances given by the software tool.

4.3   Diet Tracking System

Many dietary management software tools for CKD have a diet tracking system and a food database. The diet tracking system allows the user to enter keywords into a search box to retrieve a list of food items having these keywords. The user selects an item from the list, enters the portion size, and adds it into the food diary. Based on the items in the food diary, the diet tracking system calculates the diet's nutritional components and compares them to the allowances produced by the software tool, in a way similar to what dietitians do when providing nutrition therapy.

On their food information page, some dietary management software tools for CKD code certain nutrients in different colors to indicate whether these nutrients exceed the user's daily allowances. For example, green means that the user's intake for a specific nutrient is within the user's allowance. Red means that the user's intake for a specific nutrient is near or over the user's allowance for that day. Some dietary management software tools for CKD provide a kidney-friendly score for each food item based on its overall nutrition composition. A high score means that the food item is safe for kidneys. A low score means that the food item should be avoided or consumed in small quantity. For example, a food item high in phosphorus can be given a low score, warning users that the food item is not good for their kidneys. This helps users adjust their eating behaviors.

4.4   Diet Recommender System

Some dietary management software tools for CKD translate nutrient allowances into meal choices by generating food combinations as close to these allowances as possible in addition to displaying the values of these allowances. For example, a CKD patient can find it difficult to adhere to a dietary phosphorus limit of <1200 mg/day. While the diet tracking system can indicate that certain food items are high in phosphorus, the user may not know which food items are available as alternatives to help control his phosphorus intake. In this case, the diet recommender system can generate a complete, kidney-friendly meal plan that considers the user's dietary phosphorus limit to help him reach his nutritional goal.

5   Open Issues and Potential Solutions

Dietary management software offers the promise of dietary self-management for CKD patients. However, existing dietary management software for CKD has several limitations. In this section, we list some open issues concerning dietary management software for CKD and propose some possible solutions.

5.1   Integration with Personal Health Records

Existing dietary management software for CKD has several shortcomings in its health data input interface. First, many existing software tools ask users to enter their health data manually. This requires labor-intensive data input and can discourage users from using the software. Second, users often lack enough medical knowledge to fully understand their health conditions and the medical terms used on the input interface. As a result, the quality of health data entered by users can be questionable. Third, many health data elements are dynamic and change over time. The user's weight can fluctuate. The user's kidney function can decline as his/her CKD progresses. Lab test results typically change on a daily basis. Thus, the database storing the user's health data needs to be updated regularly.

To overcome these shortcomings and obtain more up-to-date health data of users, the dietary management software for CKD can be integrated with personal health records. This improves the dietary management software's usability, as (1) users no longer need to input their health data and (2) this ensures data accuracy and that the most up-to-date health data are used for generating dietary recommendations. Synchronizing the dietary management software with personal health records means connecting with healthcare providers with a two-way flow of information. The dietary management software is updated with users' current clinical data. The healthcare providers' information systems can be updated with information on users' nutritional status, dietary habits, and general well-being. To perform this integration, we need to develop and implement appropriate data and messaging standards for nutrition and dietary domains to support interoperability with different personal health records. With appropriate approvals, a data store from such an integration can be repurposed for further biomedical research on CKD and nutrition.

5.2   Diet Tracking System

Many dietary management software tools for CKD include a search tool for locating desired food items from a nutrition database, such as the one developed by the United States Department of Agriculture [17]. However, many of these software tools received poor ratings on the Apple and Android app stores, as users find that the diet tracking system has limited options for inputting dietary data and is cumbersome to use. Users are required to record their dietary intake each time they eat something. This is time-consuming and labor-intensive, causing users to lose patience. Moreover, the food search and data entry processes require experience with computers and can be challenging for the elderly or patients with low education levels. Since CKD is more prevalent in the elderly [18], the diet tracking system need to be senior-friendly and provide an easier and faster approach for inputting dietary data.

To make the dietary data input system more user-friendly, several new features can be added to dietary management software for CKD. Example features include a built-in barcode scanner, photo reminder, expanded database with new food products and restaurant food, allowing users to create their own recipes, saving users' favorite food combinations, and providing an option to add food items often consumed together, such as bread and butter. Some users consider a category look-up method easier to use than the traditional search method. Besides the search function, users can be given an option to click on multi-layered food category menus to locate common food items. For example, a user can click the fruit category and then the apple category to locate gala apple in the food database.

5.3   Food Sources

Nutrition information is not limited to calories and nutrient compositions. Sometimes, the food source matters. For example, proteins from plant sources are more protective of kidneys than proteins from animal sources [19]. As another example, food additives (e.g., sodium phosphate) are widely used in preparing processed foods including cheese, meat, beverages, and baked products. Phosphorus from food additives is absorbed almost completely by the human digestive tract. In comparison, only 60 % of phosphorus from natural sources is absorbed [20]. Thus, phosphorus from food additives is more problematic for CKD patients than phosphorus from natural sources. Most dietary management software tools for CKD focus on nutrient compositions and overlook food sources essential for a healthy diet. Ideally, when producing the kidney-friendly score for a specific food item, the dietary management software needs to consider the food source in addition to calculating the nutrient composition. In this way, evidence-based nutrition knowledge can be better used.

5.4   Nutrition Facts Labels

The Food and Drug Administration requires a nutrition facts label to be included on most food packages. The nutrition facts label must detail the levels of several nutrients such as cholesterol, sodium, sugar, and protein. However, no law requires phosphorus or potassium to be listed on the nutrition facts label. Thus, phosphorus and potassium levels are usually omitted from the food databases in diet tracking systems. This causes dietary management software to often underestimate a user's dietary intake of phosphorus and potassium, which needs to be closely monitored for CKD patients.

Given limited resources, it would be difficult to analyze the phosphorus and potassium levels of each food item and to update the food database manually. Nevertheless, there are several other ways to keep track of phosphorus and potassium. First, certain ingredients of processed food can be included in the food database. As mentioned earlier, CKD patients need to avoid food containing phosphorus additives. Food additives, including those containing phosphorus, are required by law to be listed on food ingredient labels. The diet tracking system can include phosphorus additives in the food database and warn users of their presence. Second, the diet tracking system can automatically issue a warning for whole food naturally high in phosphorus or potassium, if their values are missing from the nutrition facts label. For example, banana, yogurt, and potatoes are high potassium food (i.e., more than 200 mg of potassium per serving). If their potassium values are missing from the nutrition facts label, the diet tracking system can automatically identify them and give the user a warning.

5.5   Medications and Dietary Supplements

Certain medications and dietary supplements can affect overall nutrition levels, but are ignored by existing dietary management software tools for CKD. For example, some medications and dietary supplements contain high levels of phosphorus. As another example, phosphorus binders are medications that reduce the gastrointestinal tract's absorption rate of phosphates and greatly influence a patient's phosphorus level. Dietary management software for CKD needs to consider these medications and dietary supplements when producing dietary recommendations.

5.6   Nutrition Education

Most dietary management software tools for CKD assume that users have at least some knowledge about CKD and nutrition, and provide no additional information beyond a nutritional goal. However, many users, especially those with newly diagnosed CKD, are unfamiliar with CKD. Even if they have nutritional goals, they do not know how to change their diets to achieve these goals. By providing concrete examples of what they can eat, a dietary management software tool can be more useful for them. For example, the software tool can suggest a user to limit his/her protein intake to less than 80 g per day. However, with no background in nutrition, the user has no idea what 80 g of protein look like. In this case, the software tool can provide some concrete examples such as "You will consume 80 g of protein if you eat 2 eggs, 4 oz of lean fish, 4 oz of lean beef, 1/2 cup of tofu, and 1 cup of milk."

CKD self-management education can improve clinical outcomes [21]. Nutrition education tends to be more effective when actionable strategies are made explicit to help people achieve their targeted behaviors [22]. The dietary management software for CKD can educate patients about why their lab test results matter, common food sources, vital nutrients, and how to estimate portion sizes and read nutrition facts labels. For example, patients with stage 4 CKD and high serum potassium levels would benefit from education about common foods high in potassium that need to be avoided. A Web-based dietary management software tool can display education materials in a text box when the user positions the cursor on a relevant term.

Ideally, a dietary management software tool for CKD should personalize patient education based on the patient's specific needs. For example, some CKD patients need to follow a diet high in protein and low in phosphorus. Most high protein foods (e.g., meat and eggs) are also high in phosphorus. This makes it difficult for patients to adhere to appropriate diet. In this case, the dietary management software can give users tips on increasing their protein intake without over-consuming phosphorus. Examples of such tips include avoiding organ and processed meat, choosing non-enriched rice milk instead of regular milk, and consuming vegetable protein rather than animal protein.

5.7   Sharing Meal Plans

Some CKD patients need to follow a highly restricted diet, making it difficult for them to find foods they enjoy eating. For example, consider stage-4 CKD patients who also have hypertension and high serum potassium and phosphorus levels. To reduce damage to their kidneys and avoid various complications, these patients need to follow a diet low in proteins, phosphorus, sodium, and potassium. Their dietitians may have given them a long list of food items that they should avoid. This list informs them what they cannot eat, but not what they can eat. With all the restrictions, these patients can have difficulty finding foods they enjoy. Hence, they often completely abandon their diets.

To address this issue, the diet recommender system can automatically generate food combinations meeting the patient's nutritional goals. For example, the dietary management software tool can check each recipe in its database against all dietary restrictions. However, having too many restrictions can prevent the software tool from finding a solution acceptable to the user. To solve this problem, the software tool can allow patients to share their food diary or meal plans with those having similar dietary restrictions. By communicating with each other, patients can find new cookbooks and recipes giving more dietary options.

5.8   Evaluation of Dietary Management Software for CKD

To our best knowledge, no research has been published evaluating dietary management software for CKD. Existing dietary management software tools for CKD vary in their development process, theoretical framework, and knowledge base accuracy. To provide high-quality health information, qualified healthcare professionals including nephrologists, dietitians, and nutritionists should be involved in compiling and reviewing knowledge stored in the knowledge base. Also, the dietary management software tool's efficacy should be evaluated through controlled clinical trials with CKD patients.

5.9 Senior-Friendly User Interface

A major issue in using health information technology for dietary management among CKD patients is the digital divide. The digital divide refers to the economic or social gap between those who have access to modern technologies and those who do not or are unaware of them. CKD is correlated with old age and low socioeconomic status [18]. When developing a dietary management software tool for CKD, the developer needs to consider the fact that many users will have little experience with computers. The software tool's graphical user interface needs to be senior-friendly and intuitive. Also, mobile apps for CKD patients need to include an option for larger fonts, adjustable contrast, and an interface with simple prompts such as "yes" and "no."

6 Conclusion

Computer-based interventions can be cost-effective if they can reach sufficiently large populations and confer discernable health benefits [23]. Using medical knowledge to automatically provide users with personalized nutrition care, dietary management software holds great promise for improving health and reducing costs for CKD patients. This paper provides an overview of existing dietary management software for CKD and identifies several open issues. In addition, we propose some possible solutions to these open issues in the hope of benefiting future research.

References

1. Vassalotti, J.A., Centor, R., Turner, B.J., Greer, R.C., Choi, M., Sequist, T.D.: National Kidney Foundation Kidney Disease Outcomes Quality Initiative: practical approach to detection and management of chronic kidney disease for the primary care clinician. Am. J. Med. **129**(2), 153–162.e7 (2016)
2. National Kidney Foundation: K/DOQI clinical practice guidelines for chronic kidney disease: evaluation, classification, and stratification. Am. J. Kidney Dis. **39**(2), S1–S266 (2002)
3. KDIGO: KDIGO 2012 clinical practice guideline for the evaluation and management of chronic kidney disease. Kidney Int. Suppl. **3**(1), 1–150 (2013)
4. USRDS: United States Renal Data System 2015 annual data report, Chap. 6: Medicare expenditures for persons with CKD (2015). http://www.usrds.org/2015/view/v1_06.aspx
5. Fouque, D., Pelletier, S., Mafra, D., Chauveau, P.: Nutrition and chronic kidney disease. Kidney Int. **80**(4), 348–357 (2011)

6. Wright Nunes, J.A., Wallston, K.A., Eden, S.K., Shintani, A.K., Ikizler, T.A., Cavanaugh, K.L.: Associations among perceived and objective disease knowledge and satisfaction with physician communication in patients with chronic kidney disease. Kidney Int. **80**(12), 1344–1351 (2011)
7. USRDS: United States Renal Data System 2010 Annual Data Report, Healthy People 2010 (2010). http://www.usrds.org/2010/pdf/v2_00hp.pdf
8. Cho, M.E., Beddhu, S.: Dietary recommendations for patients with nondialysis CKD (2016). http://www.uptodate.com/contents/dietary-recommendations-for-patients-with-nondialysis-ckd
9. Institute of Medicine: Dietary Reference Intakes for Energy, Carbohydrate, Fiber, Fat, Fatty Acids, Cholesterol, Protein, and Amino Acids, pp. 589–768. The National Academies Press, Washington DC (2005)
10. Chen, X., Beddhu, S.: Nutrition and chronic kidney disease. In: Bales, C.W., Locher, J.L., Saltzman, E. (eds.) Handbook of Clinical Nutrition and Aging, 3rd edn, pp. 261–271. Springer, New York (2015)
11. Brug, J., Oenema, A., Campbell, M.: Past, present, and future of computer-tailored nutrition education. Am. J. Clin. Nutr. **77**(4 Suppl), 1028S–1034S (2003)
12. Kipnis, V., Subar, A.F., Midthune, D., Freedman, L.S., Ballard-Barbash, R., Troiano, R.P., Bingham, S., Schoeller, D.A., Schatzkin, A., Carroll, R.J.: Structure of dietary measurement error: results of the OPEN biomarker study. Am. J. Epidemiol. **158**(1), 14–21 (2003)
13. Carter, M.C., Burley, V.J., Nykjaer, C., Cade, J.E.: 'My Meal Mate' (MMM): validation of the diet measures captured on a smartphone application to facilitate weight loss. Br. J. Nutr. **109**(3), 539–546 (2013)
14. Carter, M.C., Burley, V.J., Nykjaer, C., Cade, J.E.: Adherence to a smartphone application for weight loss compared to website and paper diary: pilot randomized controlled trial. J. Med. Internet Res. **15**(4), e32 (2013)
15. Skouroliakou, M., Kakavelaki, C., Diamantopoulos, K., Stathopoulou, M., Vourvouhaki, E., Souliotis, K.: The development and implementation of a software tool and its effect on the quality of provided clinical nutritional therapy in hospitalized patients. J. Am. Med. Inform. Assoc. **16**(6), 802–805 (2009)
16. Hong, S.M., Cho, J.Y., Lee, J.H., Kim, G., Kim, M.C.: NutriSonic web expert system for meal management and nutrition counseling with nutrient time-series analysis, e-food exchange and easy data transition. Nutr. Res. Pract. **2**(2), 121–129 (2008)
17. NDL/FNIC food composition database homepage (2016). http://ndb.nal.usda.gov/
18. Diamantidis, C.J., Becker, S.: Health information technology (IT) to improve the care of patients with chronic kidney disease (CKD). BMC Nephrol. **15**, 7 (2014)
19. Chen, X., Wei, G., Jalili, T., Metos, J., Giri, A., Cho, M.E., Boucher, R., Greene, T., Beddhu, S.: The associations of plant protein intake with all-cause mortality in CKD. Am. J. Kidney Dis. **67**(3), 423–430 (2015)
20. Uribarri, J., Calvo, M.S.: Hidden sources of phosphorus in the typical American diet: does it matter in nephrology? Semin. Dial. **16**(3), 186–188 (2003)
21. Enworom, C.D., Tabi, M.: Evaluation of kidney disease education on clinical outcomes and knowledge of self-management behaviors of patients with chronic kidney disease. Nephrol Nurs. J. **42**(4), 363–372 (2015)
22. Contento, I.R.: Nutrition education: linking research, theory, and practice. Asia Pac. J. Clin. Nutr. **17**(Suppl 1), 176–179 (2008)
23. Booth, A.O., Nowson, C.A., Matters, H.: Evaluation of an interactive, Internet-based weight loss program: a pilot study. Health Educ. Res. **23**(3), 371–381 (2008)

EQClinic: A Platform for Improving Medical Students' Clinical Communication Skills

Chunfeng Liu[1], Rafael A. Calvo[1(✉)], Renee Lim[1,2], and Silas Taylor[3]

[1] School of Electrical and Information Engineering,
The University of Sydney, Sydney, Australia
{chunfeng.liu, rafael.calvo, renee.lim}@sydney.edu.au
[2] Sydney Medical School, The University of Sydney, Sydney, Australia
[3] UNSW Medicine, UNSW Australia, Sydney, Australia
silas.taylor@unsw.edu.au

Abstract. Communication is important in clinical interaction; thus medical students require communication skills training. Most training programs focus on developing students' verbal skills, and nonverbal communication is not given sufficient attention. This paper describes a tele-health training platform EQClinic, which has the capability of automatically detecting nonverbal behaviour in tele-consultations and providing medical students with human and computer-generated feedback for improving their communication skills. In this paper, we describe EQClinic's components and report preliminary results from an 8-week user study with 135 medical students. The students were provided two opportunities of having face-to-face consultation, and between these two consultations students were also asked to complete a tele-consultation using EQClinic. Student found the system usable and their scores in the second face-to-face consultations improved after the tele-consultation (from 12.58 to 13.53, p = 0.005). The results suggest that EQClinic positively influenced medical students' learning and may be a valuable tool in medical education.

1 Introduction

Efficient patient-clinician communication can lead to better health outcomes [16]. As the medical education community has realized the importance of clinical communication, more training programs have been offered for students to learn clinical communication skills. Providing medical students with video recording feedback is a traditional training method in clinical communication skills teaching [2]. Medical students reported benefiting from reviewing videotapes of their clinical consultations with real or *simulated* patients (e.g. actors or trained volunteers) [13] especially when observers' feedback about students' verbal or nonverbal behaviours were also provided with the video recordings [2]. Most training programs focus on verbal communication, while nonverbal communication which is the major communication channel [5] is not given sufficient attention. Providing manually annotated nonverbal behaviour feedback is a common way to enhance nonverbal communication skill learning [7]. However, this method is too time-consuming to be widely adopted in the teaching curriculum.

© Springer International Publishing AG 2016
X. Yin et al. (Eds.): HIS 2016, LNCS 10038, pp. 73–84, 2016.
DOI: 10.1007/978-3-319-48335-1_8

The dramatic improvement in behaviour recognition techniques in the computer sciences [17], has led to the development of applications that are able to automatically detect nonverbal behaviour. For example, Hoque et al. [6] developed a social skills training platform that allowed users to communicate with a virtual actor, and was able to automatically sense the nonverbal behaviours of the user. After the conversation, the platform analyses the nonverbal behaviours and provides feedback for the user. However, few studies have applied these behaviour recognition techniques to medical education applications.

In this paper, we contribute a new clinical communication skills training platform EQClinic with the capability of automatically identifying nonverbal behaviours of participants in a tele-consultation. The aims of EQClinic are: (1) providing students with opportunities to communicate with simulated patients (SPs) through a tele-conference platform; (2) providing students with different forms of feedback, including video recording, assessments and comments from SPs; (3) automatically identifying students' nonverbal behaviour using computer vision and audio processing techniques, and providing graphical representations of these behaviours for students. In this paper, the main research question we address is whether medical students' communication skills were improved through using EQClinic. We examined this question through an 8-week user study. In this study, all participated students were offered two opportunities to have face-to-face consultations with SPs. Between these two consultations, all students were asked to finish a tele-consultation using EQClinic.

In this paper, we describe the main components of EQClinic (Sect. 2) and algorithms used to detect nonverbal behaviour (Sect. 3). In Sects. 4 and 5, we describe the user study design and the findings from the study. Section 6 is the general conclusions from this research.

2   EQClinic Platform

EQClinic [10] was developed by the Positive Computing lab at the University of Sydney Australia in collaboration with medical schools at the University of Sydney and the University of New South Wales (UNSW) Australia. Figure 1 illustrates the five main components of EQClinic, which are an online training component, a personal calendar, a real-time interaction component, a nonverbal behaviour detector and a feedback generator. In the following sections, we separately describe each of these components.

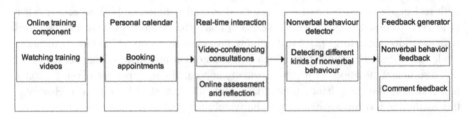

Fig. 1. System architecture of EQClinic

Training component and personal calendar: EQClinic provides a training component for students and SPs to familiarize themselves with the platform. Training videos and documents are provided in this component to guide the users. EQClinic also provides students and SPs with an automated personal calendar. SPs can offer their available time slots on the calendar to allow students to make a booking. Emails and SMS notifications are sent from the platform when users request and confirm appointments.

Real-time interaction component: After the appointment has been confirmed, students and SPs can have tele-consultations through the real-time interaction component. This component includes the video conferencing component and online assessments. The video conferencing component works on most web browsers of a PC or an Android tablet. Once both participants are connected, the system automatically records the consultation. This component uses OpenTok, a Web Real-Time Communication (WebRTC) service, to provide real time video communication. EQClinic also provides SPs with two tools: a thumbs tool, which provides a simple tool for SPs to indicate positive (thumbs up) and negative (thumbs down) moments during the consultation, and a comments box. Both forms of feedback are stored with timestamps and can be seen by the students when they review the consultation recording. The students' video conferencing page is similar to the SPs' except that the two tools are not included.

In order to facilitate the learning through reflection process for students, we developed online assessment interactions, where SPs evaluate the performance of the students through an assessment form immediately after the tele-consultation. The students also conduct a self-assessment, and reflect on their tele-consultation. When the SP finishes the assessment form, the results can be reviewed by the student immediately and the student can comment on the assessment. Answering these reflective questions is compulsory for students.

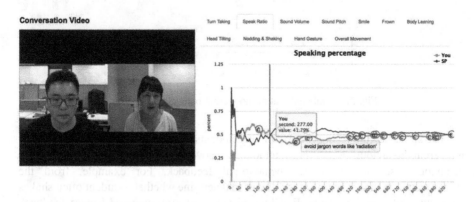

Fig. 2. Single-feature nonverbal behaviours feedback

Nonverbal behaviour detector: When the tele-consultation is completed, EQClinic automatically analyses the video recordings using audio processing and computer vision techniques. The system mainly detects the following types of nonverbal behaviour: head movements (nodding, head shaking and head tilting), facial expressions (smiling and frowning), body movements (body leaning and overall body movements), voice properties (volume and pitch) and speech patterns (turn taking and speaking ratio changes). Each 15-min video recording takes around 55 min to be analysed on a personal computer with 3.40 GHz CPU and 16 GB RAM. The details of the algorithms that are used in EQClinic for detecting these behaviours will be introduced in Sect. 3.

Feedback generator: A single-feature feedback report illustrates each form of nonverbal behaviour separately. Figure 2 is an example of a single-feature feedback report that describes the speaking ratio of the student. Comments (the "C" labels) from the SP are also show on the graphs. On clicking a point on the graph, the video moves to that particular timestamp. With this report, students can easily observe variations of a particular nonverbal behaviour during a consultation.

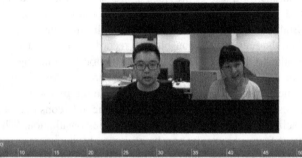

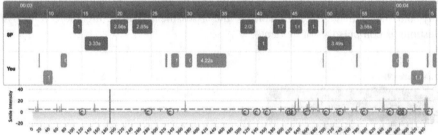

Fig. 3. Combined-feature nonverbal behaviours feedback

The single-feature feedback report helps students to focus on a single aspect of their nonverbal behaviour. However, interactions between different types of nonverbal behaviour also provide useful behavioural feedback. For example, from the single-feature feedback report, it is difficult to determine whether a student often shakes his head while smiling. Thus, EQClinic also provides a combined-feature feedback report that displays multiple kinds of nonverbal behaviour on one page (turn-taking and smile intensity in Fig. 3). Students are able to combine different types of nonverbal behaviour according to their needs.

3 Nonverbal Behaviour Detection

EQClinic detects five categories of nonverbal behaviours. This decision was based on a combination of knowledge regarding nonverbal behaviours in previous clinical consultation literature and the capability of current technology to detect these behaviours. In the following sections, we describe details of the algorithms we adopted for detecting nonverbal behaviours.

Head movements: EQClinic detects three kinds of head movements: nodding, head shaking and head tilting. The fundamental procedure of detecting head movements is identifying the landmarks of a face. ASMLibrary [19], which is able to locate 68 facial landmarks, is adopted by EQClinic.

EQClinic senses nodding and head shaking by tracking the mid-point between the two inner corners of the eyes [9]. Using this method, every frame of the video recording can be classified into one of three states: stable state, extreme state and transient state. If there are more than two extreme states between the current and the previous stable frames, and all adjacent extreme frames differ by more than two pixels in the x coordinate, then the algorithm assumes that a head shaking has occurred. Head nodding and head shaking are similar movements for this algorithm, except that nodding appears in the y axis.

After locating the landmarks, it is easy to calculate the tilting angle of the head. Tilting angle is represented as the angle between the vertical line and the line contains the tip of node point and the mid-point.

Facial expression: EQClinic detects two kinds of facial expression: smiling and frowning. Training and classifying steps was included on detecting smiles. In the training step, 100 smile images and 100 non-smile images from the GENKI4 K dataset [4] were selected as the training set. Firstly, the detector extracted the mouth areas of training images using Haar-cascade classifier provided by OpenCV [18], and then regulated the size of each extracted area as 100 * 70 pixels. In the classifying step, Principal Components Analysis (PCA) is used to classify images [15]. By comparing an image with the training set, the algorithm identifies whether this image contains a smile expression. 69 smile and 585 non-smile images which included in the CK+ dataset [11] were selected to evaluate the accuracy of the smile detection algorithm. The precision, recall and F1-score of this algorithm were 0.78, 0.96 and 0.86 respectively.

In order to test frowning, three steps need to be performed. The first step is locating the landmarks of a face. Then the detector extracts the area between the two eyebrows. Lastly, the detector processes the extracted area using SOBEL filter and classifies whether the image contains frowning [1]. The processed image which contains more than 1% white pixels is considered a frown image [1]. 38 frown images (from the anger category) and 38 non-frown images (from the neutral category) were selected from CK + dataset [11] to evaluate the accuracy of this algorithm. These images were gathered from 38 different people, and each person contributed one frown image and one non-frown image. As a result, the precision, recall and F1-score of this algorithm were 0.79, 0.71 and 0.75 respectively.

Body movements: EQClinic detects two kinds of body movements: body leaning and overall body movements. EQClinic detects body leaning by observing the changes of the face size. When the size of the face dramatically increases, a forward body leaning has happened. Similarly, a backward leaning has happened when the size of the face decreases. Overall body movement detection does not focus on a particular kind of movement. It represents the overall level of the participant's body movements. The core idea of this detection is calculating the difference in pixels between every adjacent pair of video frames [3]. The higher the value is, the more dramatically the participant moves.

Voice properties and speech pattern: The volume and sound pitch are the two voice properties detected by EQClinic. An open source Matlab library was adopted by EQClinic to detect these properties [8]. EQClinic represents the volume in decibels (db) and represents the sound pitch in Semitones. EQClinic detects two kinds of speech pattern: turn-taking and speaking ratio. Turn taking illustrates all the speaking and silence periods of both participants. EQClinic also concludes the longest speaking period and average length of each speaking turn. Speaking ratio describes the cumulative percentage of total time the student and the SP each spoke within a given time frame. A key procedure of detecting these two features is End Point Detection (EPD). The aim of EPD is to identify the start and end point of an audio segment. A time domain method, which contains a volume threshold and a zero crossing rate, is used for EPD [8].

4 Pilot User Study

4.1 Participants

Participants were 83 volunteer/actor simulated patients, 28 tutors of clinical communication skill and 135 Year-2 medical students from an Australian medical school. All students were enrolled in a communication skills training course provided by the medical school. This study was approved by UNSW Research Committee (HC Reference Number: HC16048).

4.2 Instruments

Five questionnaires were used in the study. The Pre-interview and Post-interview Questionnaire examined students' understanding of communication skills. Five questions (three 7-point scale Likert and two free-text questions) were included in these two questionnaires:

1. How confident do you feel now about your communication skills?
2. Do nonverbal behaviours have a significant effect on medical communication?
3. Is verbal content the main factor that affects medical communication?
4. What do you think are the three main nonverbal behaviours that affect medical communication?
5. Are there any specific communication skills you would like to work on?

In addition, Post-interview Questionnaire also included some questions to evaluate the system usability. The Post-interview Nonverbal Behaviour Reflection Questionnaire asked students to estimate how often they engaged in certain nonverbal behaviours during the interview. Reflection Questionnaire aimed to help students to reflect on the consultation. Student-Patient Observed Communication Assessment (SOCA) Form was used to assess students' communication skills. It was an edited version of the Calgary Cambridge Guide [14], and evaluated students' communication skills from four aspects on a four-point scale: providing structures, gathering information, building rapport and understanding the patient's needs.

4.3   Study Design and Procedure

The study started from April of 2016 and last for 8 weeks. Three phases were included in this study. In weeks 1 and 2, students completed a face-to-face consultation with SPs. Then, from weeks 3 to 6, all students were asked to finish a tele-consultation using EQClinic. Lastly, in weeks 7 and 8, students completed another face-to-face consultation. In this study, having two face-to-face consultations was not compulsory, but finishing an EQClinic practice was mandatory for each student. All consultations focused on history taking, to ensure a structured and consistent interaction.

Tele-consultations: Volunteer/actor SPs were recruited through emails, and asked to complete the online training and provide availabilities on their EQClinic calendar. In the SPs' online training component, a patient scenario was provided. The scenario mentioned the main symptoms for the patient to present and included having intermittent chest pain and an unproductive cough for 5 days. All SPs had previous experience in simulated face-to-face consultations; therefore we did not provide them with separate training on performance.

Students were requested, by email, to complete one tele-consultation with a SP through EQClinic. The email described the details of the study and asked them to log into EQClinic to watch the training videos. It also informed them that once they completed the training, they could request a consultation time from the slots available on their personal calendar. The SPs and students were allowed to have the tele-consultation anywhere as long as there was: (1) A web browser on a PC or an Android tablet with external or build-in camera and microphone; (2) A good Internet connection; (3) Good lighting.

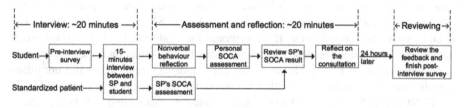

Fig. 4. Workflow of having an EQClinic consultation

We divided each tele-consultation into three parts: interviewing, assessing and reviewing (Fig. 4). The interview and assessment components took around 40 min for a student and 25–30 min for a SP to complete. In the interviewing section, the student filled out the Pre-interview Questionnaire and then the student and the SP had a 15-min interview through the tele-conference component. In the assessing section, the student and the SP completed the online assessments. After each interview, the SP assessed the performance of the student using the SOCA Form. The student estimated their non-verbal behaviour using the Post Interview Nonverbal Behaviour Reflection Question-naire, completed a personal SOCA Form, reviewed the SP's Assessment Form and reflected on the interview using the Reflection Questionnaire.

As EQClinic took time to analyse the video and identify nonverbal behaviours, the students were emailed and asked to return to the system 24 h after the consultation to review different kinds of feedback, which included the video recording, the comments from the SP and the automated nonverbal behaviour feedback, and fill out the Post-interview Questionnaire.

Face-to-face consultations: The administrator of this study manually scheduled the face-to-face appointments. Experienced SPs were recruited through emails. No training was provided in this phase for these SPs. The face-to-face consultations were con-ducted at the simulated clinical consultation rooms of the university. Besides a student and a SP, during the consultation, a tutor was also presented in the room to observe the performance of the student. After the consultation, the tutor completed a SOCA Form to assess the student. The students were provided with the tutors' assessments to review. The SP did not provide any evaluation and feedback for the student in this phase. The scenario design and length of face-to-face consultations were same as tele-consultations.

5 Result and Discussion

135 students were participated in this study. 107 (79 %) students completed a face-to-face consultation in weeks 1 and 2. 130 (96 %) students finished the tele-consultation during weeks 3 to 6. In the last period (weeks 7 and 8), 35 students had a face-to-face consultation, and 30 of them completed a face-to-face consultation in weeks 1 and 2. Table 1 lists the mean scores of the SOCA assessments in different study periods.

As a baseline communication skills testing in weeks 1 and 2, students (n = 107) achieved 12.58 average total SOCA score. After having a tele-consultation using EQClinic, their mean score significantly increased to 13.53 (n = 30, p = 0.005) in the second face-to-face consultation. If we explored the students (n = 13) who reviewed the nonverbal behaviour feedback which provided by EQClinic, their mean score was even higher (mean = 13.62). However, these 13 students' mean scores did not differ from the students who did not complete the nonverbal feedback review (mean = 13.47, n = 17/30, p > 0.05). This result would seem to indicate that having EQClinic practice and reviewing nonverbal behaviour feedback improved the students' communication skills. 43 % (13/30) of the students reviewed the nonverbal behaviour feedback, and

Table 1. Mean SOCA scores (SOCA total score was on range 4–16, F2F-Con2* = students who completed two face-to-face consultations, F2F-NVB* = students who completed two face-to-face consultations and reviewed the EQClinic nonverbal behaviour feedback)

Period	Week 1~2	Week 3~6	Week 7~8		
Type	F2F-Con	Tele-Con	F2F-Con	F2F-Con2*	F2F-NVB*
n	107	130	35	30	13
Providing structures	3.12 (SD = 0.53)	3.31 (SD = 0.67)	3.31 (SD = 0.52)	3.37 (SD = 0.48)	3.38 (SD = 0.49)
Gathering information	3.07 (SD = 0.56)	3.34 (SD = 0.72)	3.51 (SD = 0.55)	3.53 (SD = 0.50)	3.46 (SD = 0.50)
Building rapport	3.24 (SD = 0.56)	3.16 (SD = 0.73)	3.34 (SD = 0.58)	3.37 (SD = 0.55)	3.46 (SD = 0.63)
Understand patient's needs	3.14 (SD = 0.61)	3.32 (SD = 0.68)	3.26 (SD = 0.44)	3.27 (SD = 0.44)	3.31 (SD = 0.46)
Total score	12.58 (SD = 1.61)	13.13 (SD = 2.31)	13.43 (SD = 1.63)	13.53 (SD = 1.52)	13.62 (SD = 1.64)

this participating rate was relatively low. Improving students' engagement would be our future work. Another point we could not ignore when interpreting the result was that, after finishing the first face-to-face consultation, the students were also provided with the tutors' SOCA assessments to review. Thus, the first face-to-face practice and the assessment feedback might also contribute to the significant improvement in their second face-to-face consultation.

As mentioned in a previous study [12], compared with face-to-face consultations, students achieved lower communication skills assessment results in tele-consultation. In this study, we did not observe obvious evidences to support this statement. However, from students' free-text feedback, their performance was influenced in tele-consultations. Some students described that they found it difficult to present nonverbal behaviours, and this made it hard to build rapport with the SP. Some of them found maintaining eye-contact with patients was difficult because they could not physically look at their eyes. Students were confused about where they should look during the consultation: the middle of the screen or the camera. In addition, some students mentioned that they were unable to observe some nonverbal behaviours of the SP as only the upper-body of the SP could be seen by the student. For example, one student mentioned that "As a student, I found it difficult to gain any real sense of eye contact or other forms of non-verbal communication - only the shoulders and head were visible and eye contact was almost impossible."

Table 2 compared the results between Pre- and Post-interview Questionnaires in tele-consultations. In total, 130 students completed the Pre-interview Questionnaire and 80 students (61.5 % = 80/130) completed the Post-interview Questionnaire. Firstly, in both questionnaires, students agreed significantly more on the statements of "Nonverbal behaviours have a significant effect on medical communication" (nonverbal statement) than "Verbal content is the main factor that affects medical communication" (verbal statement) ($p < 0.0001$). These results indicated that students had realized the importance of nonverbal behaviours. In addition, 45 % of students reported that they would like to improve some communication skills related to nonverbal behaviours in the Post-interview Questionnaires, and this figure was only 23.8 % in the Pre-interview Questionnaire. This result was consistent with our previous study [10], which showed that EQClinic and its nonverbal behaviour feedback enhanced the students' awareness of nonverbal communication. As nonverbal behaviour is often performed unconsciously, understanding its importance and increasing students' awareness of it would be helpful for students to develop their communication skills.

Although on average students reported higher score of confidence about their communication skills in Post-interview Questionnaire (increased from 4.75 to 4.95), the difference was not significant ($p = 0.062$). In both questionnaires, the most students rated their confidence at 5 score ($73/130 = 56.2\%$ in Pre, $36/80 = 45\%$ in Post). In addition, we found that increased percentage of students rated their confidence at 6 score ($14/130 = 10.8\%$ in Pre, $18/80 = 22.5\%$ in Post).

Table 2 also describes students' answers related to system usability. The students felt the information (5.11/7) and structure (5.14/7) of the system were clear. However, the platform had a large space to improve on user interface design and proving appropriate feedback when users encounter errors. According to some students' text feedback, we found that some technical issues might affect the usability. The stableness

Table 2. Results of Pre- and Post-Questionnaires (all questions were in a 7-point scale, NVB* = number of students who explicitly mentioned nonverbal behaviour when answering this question)

Questions	Pre-ques	Post-ques	p
n	130	80	
How confident do you feel now about your communication skills?	4.75 (SD = 0.68)	4.95 (SD = 0.80)	0.062
Are there any specific communication skills you would like to work on? (NVB*)	31 (23.8%)	36 (45%)	
Do nonverbal behaviours have a significant effect on medical communication?	6.06 (SD = 1.26)	6.15 (SD = 0.90)	0.555
Is verbal content the main factor that affects medical communication?	4.45 (SD = 1.27)	4.76 (SD = 1.14)	0.065

Usability questions (in Post-interview Questionnaire)	Score
n	80
I feel comfortable using the system	4.68 (SD = 1.45)
The information provided with this system is clear	5.11 (SD = 1.23)
The structure of this system is clear	5.14 (SD = 1.17)
I like using the interface of this system	4.34 (SD = 1.54)
Whenever I make a mistake using this system, the system made it easy to get back to where I wanted	4.40 (SD = 1.21)

of the network was the main concern of the students. 38 (29.2 %) students reported that they experienced different levels of network interruption during the consultations. Some students missed important parts of the conversation with the SP because of the interruption of the video conferencing. Video or sound lags also bothered the students, and contributed to inappropriate interruptions of the SP.

Several limitations should be considered in our study. Firstly, futures studies should include a control group to compare, for example a group of students who did not exposure to EQClinic. However, in this study, due to requirements of the teaching curriculum, all students were asked to have an EQClinic practise. Secondly, completing two face-to-face consultations was not compulsory task for students in this study; therefore we observed increased drop-out as the semester progressed. In addition, the limited consultation scenario could not comprehensively examine students' communication skills. Lastly, all participated students in this study were junior students with limited communication skills knowledge. In order to explore the usefulness of this learning tool, senior students should also be tested on the platform.

6 Conclusion

In conclusion, this study provides an evident trend showing that providing students opportunities for tele-consultation with SPs, and offering different kinds of feedback information for students to facilitate their reflection, improved students' learning of communication skills.

This study indicated that EQClinic is a useful and practical communication skills learning tool for medical students within university settings. However, according to the current results, we are unable to determine which learning component is the most useful component to enhance students' learning. In the future, we will conduct a more detailed study to investigate this question. In addition, the growth of collected student data by EQClinic will aid the development of some rules and models using machine learning algorithms to indicate to students what nonverbal behaviour is good or bad in their clinical tele-consultations.

Acknowledgements. This project was funded by an internal grant from the Brain and Mind Centre at the University of Sydney, Australia and Australian Government. RC is funded by the Australian Research Council.

References

1. Chung, S.C., Barma, S., Kuan, T.-W., Lin, T.-W.: Frowning expression detection based on SOBEL filter for negative emotion recognition. In: 2014 IEEE International Conference on Paper Presented at the Orange Technologies (ICOT), Xi'an (2014)
2. Fukkink, R.G., Trienekens, N., Kramer, L.J.: Video feedback in education and training: Putting learning in the picture. Educ. Psychol. Rev. **23**(1), 45–63 (2011)

3. Fung, M., Jin, Y., Zhao, R., Hoque, M.E.: ROC speak: semi-automated personalized feedback on nonverbal behavior from recorded videos. In: Paper Presented at the Proceedings of the 2015 ACM International Joint Conference on Pervasive and Ubiquitous Computing, Osaka (2015)

4. GENKI-4 K: The MPLab GENKI Database, GENKI-4 K Subset. http://mplab.ucsd.edu

5. Gorawara-Bhat, R., Cook, M.A., Sachs, G.A.: Nonverbal communication in doctor–elderly patient transactions (NDEPT): development of a tool. Patient Educ. Couns. **66**(2), 223–234 (2007)

6. Hoque, M.E., Courgeon, M., Martin, J.-C., Mutlu, B., Picard, R.W.: Mach: my automated conversation coach. In: Paper Presented at the Proceedings of the 2013 ACM International Joint Conference on Pervasive and Ubiquitous Computing, Zurich (2013)

7. Ishikawa, H., Hashimoto, H., Kinoshita, M., Yano, E.: Can nonverbal communication skills be taught? Med. Teach. **32**(10), 860–863 (2010)

8. Jang, J.S.R.: Utility Toolbox (2016). http://mirlab.org/jang

9. Kawato, S., Ohya, J.: Real-time detection of nodding and head-shaking by directly detecting and tracking the "between-eyes". In: Fourth IEEE International Conference on Paper Presented at the Automatic Face and Gesture Recognition, 2000, Proceedings, Grenoble (2000)

10. Liu, C., Calvo, R.A., Lim, R.: Improving medical students' awareness of their nonverbal communication through automated nonverbal behavior feedback. Front. ICT **3**(11) (2016)

11. Lucey, P., Cohn, J.F., Kanade, T., Saragih, J., Ambadar, Z., Matthews, I.: The extended cohn-kanade dataset (ck+): a complete dataset for action unit and emotion-specified expression. In: 2010 IEEE Computer Society Conference on Paper Presented at the Computer Vision and Pattern Recognition Workshops (CVPRW), San Francisco (2010)

12. Novack, D.H., Cohen, D., Peitzman, S.J., Beadenkopf, S., Gracely, E., Morris, J.: A pilot test of WebOSCE: a system for assessing trainees' clinical skills via teleconference. Med. Teach. **24**(5), 483–487 (2002)

13. Paul, S., Dawson, K., Lanphear, J., Cheema, M.: Video recording feedback: a feasible and effective approach to teaching history-taking and physical examination skills in undergraduate paediatric medicine. Med. Educ. **32**(3), 332–336 (1998)

14. Simmenroth-Nayda, A., Heinemann, S., Nolte, C., Fischer, T., Himmel, W.: Psychometric properties of the Calgary Cambridge guides to assess communication skills of undergraduate medical students. Intl. J. Med. Educ. **5**, 212 (2014)

15. Smith, L.I.: A tutorial on principal components analysis. Cornell Univ. USA **51**(52), 65 (2002)

16. Stewart, M.A.: Effective physician-patient communication and health outcomes: a review. CMAJ Can. Med. Assoc. J. **152**(9), 1423 (1995)

17. Vinciarelli, A., Pantic, M., Bourlard, H.: Social signal processing: survey of an emerging domain. Image Vis. Comput. **27**(12), 1743–1759 (2009)

18. Viola, P., Jones, M.: Rapid object detection using a boosted cascade of simple features. In: Proceedings of the 2001 IEEE Computer Society Conference on Paper Presented at the Computer Vision and Pattern Recognition, 2001, CVPR 2001, Kauai (2001)

19. Wei, Y.: Research on facial expression recognition and synthesis. Master Thesis, Department of Computer Science and Technology, Nanjing (2009)

Internet Hospital: Challenges and Opportunities in China

Liwei Xu[✉]

Huizhou Medicine Institute, Huizhou, China
mrxuliwei@gmail.com

Abstract. Internet hospital via telecommunication technologies redefines the healthcare delivery concept and starts to revolutionize the traditional health sector. This new method has a significant advantage to deliver proper medical resources to the rural and remote area with less cost timely and improves rural healthcare capacity. However, quality and safety concerns have not been addressed by any reliable evidence. The internet hospital can go beyond diagnosis and treatment and find opportunities in training and education and diseases management in China.

1 Introduction

Internet hospital is a new term in China, which has attracted the attention of patients, medical practitioners and investors. At present, there is not a universal definition of internet hospital, whereas its main purpose is to reduce the rural population's difficulty in accessing to modern healthcare [1]. In China, a large proportion of the rural population is struggling to accessing to the adequate healthcare, and there is always an uneven number of people with chronic illness, especially elderly people [2, 3]. The internet hospital aims to reduce the logistic needs by enabling the rural patients to receive better healthcare in urban areas [4]. Besides, another purpose of internet hospital is to solve the overcrowded issues of outpatient hospital service caused by the lack of trust in general practitioners [5].

The internet hospital is a healthcare delivery method that enables patients to be remotely examined by physicians with information communication technologies, which is also called telemedicine in most developed and developing countries [6]. The services provided through internet hospitals include radiology, cardiology, pathology as well as remote consultation.

Internet hospital has not been commonly known until 2014, and it is a term that describes the combination of the internet industry and health industry. The internet industry in China is trying to replace the physical hospital with the internet one just like what it has done in replacing physical shops with online shops in the last 1–2 decades [7]. Investors believe that remote consultation, which means that the patients talk with doctors in clinics while sitting in their own bedrooms, is the future of healthcare [1].

X. Yin et al. (Eds.): HIS 2016, LNCS 10038, pp. 85–90, 2016.
DOI: 10.1007/978-3-319-48335-1_9

2   Need for Internet Hospital in China

As a new healthcare delivery concept in China, internet hospital will improve the healthcare capability in rural areas. China is a country with a large population, most of whom live in rural areas [8]. Unlike the urban areas that have available high-quality hospital outpatient service, rural and remote areas often have community healthcare facilities with very low medical capacity: less qualified physicians, inexperienced primary providers as well as out-of-date diagnostic equipments [2]. All of these lead to the consequences of inability to respond to emergency, late discovery of ailment, delayed treatment and rural patients' faith loss in community healthcare facilities [2]. Nevertheless, the implementation of internet hospital can create an extensive medical support network to back up the primary providers in rural areas with experts in urban regions, and then patients will have more opportunities to consult the specialists without travelling to urban hospitals [9]. In this way, the internet hospital will solve the gap between urban and rural healthcare services, promotes the accessibility to rural healthcare, improves the health outcome and reduces the transportation time and cost for rural population; thus, it is a good complement of traditional physical healthcare.

3   Internet Hospital Types

Internet hospital application is not limited to one form, and investors in various fields have built different forms of internet hospitals in China. More than hundreds of internet hospitals have been launched since the first internet hospital went online in 2014. They can be grouped into three main types: those launched by a physical hospital, launched by an internet company and the internet hospital platform.

3.1   Launched by a Physical Hospital

This type of internet hospital is launched by an existing top-level hospital, using its current physicians to provide services through telecommunication technologies. The most typical case is the Guangdong Internet Hospital, which is the first internet hospital in China and launched by Guangdong Second Hospital in 2014 [5]. It gathers the in-house spare physicians together and transfers them into a new department that dedicatedly provides remote consultation over the internet [10]. On the average, this internet hospital receives 2,500 online patients per day, and the average cost of the prescription is CNY60, a quarter of the average medicine cost of a top-level hospital outpatient service visit [11]. However, the internet hospital has not to charge the online patients consultation fees, and it plans to charge CNY10 per consultation for most general issues and chronic diseases pending government approval [5], which is considered to be reasonable in the area.

3.2   Launched by an Internet Company

This form of internet hospital is invested by the private company and is not supported by an existing hospital. It contracts directly with doctors across the country, who use their spare and leisure time to provide online consultation [12]. Wuzhen Internet Hospital is the first and biggest internet hospital practice in this business structure and model. Doctors here have the right to determine the consultation fee. However, the fee charged by its contracted doctors ranges from CNY50 to CNY1000 per 15 min [13], which is far higher than the highest consultation fee of a top hospital [11]. In consequence, the consultation has become a commercialized commodity that allows patients to compete for.

3.3 Internet Hospital of Platform Type

The internet hospital can be a platform type; it welcomes physicians or hospitals from anywhere in the country to start the practice online. The platform develops software to support physicians and patients for easy communication and streamline the registration and payment process. Ali Health, a part of Alibaba, the biggest internet company in China, has launched the first internet hospital platform on Jan 18, 2016 [7]. This practice is welcomed by the villagers in remote areas, and now they, without paying extra transportation fee, can access to better healthcare services with the same cost as the urban patients.

All these types of internet hospitals are good attempts to improve the healthcare capacity and reduce the difficulty of rural and remote population in receiving good health care service. Moreover, the development in business structure and model provides patients with various options and better medical services.

4   Economic Impact

There is no doubt that the internet reduces the traveling need of rural patients, which then lowers the transportation costs and minimize the productivity loss due to absence from work [4, 9, 14]. For the community, it increases the workload of local pharmacy and laboratory and creates more job opportunities in local area [9]; furthermore, the improvement of health outcome because of the increasing healthcare accessibility reduces local expenditure on health, and the money saved from healthcare can be allocated to other use for a higher productivity. However, according to Whitten et al.'s researches on developed and developing countries, the cost-effectiveness of tele-healthcare seems to reduce the cost of patients and providers, but it actually has not been improved because often that the costs of telecommunication infrastructure, additional personnel and management supported by government have not been taken into account [14].

5   Potential Challenges

China is experiencing a health care reform called the 3-tier healthcare system reform, which aims to increase the use of primary providers in communities and reduce the workload of outpatient hospital services and free specialists in treating mild symptoms [3]. However, most internet hospitals use specialists to serve online patients, and most of them only have common general issues such as flu, cough as well as running nose, which can be cured by family doctors in local communities. Consequently, internet hospitals compete with primary providers in specialists who are over demanded in traditional care approaches. Therefore, it goes against the central government's healthcare reform that requires common general issues to be treated by primary providers rather than specialists [3].

Other than the Wuzhen Internet Hospital, most internet hospitals are not allowed to charge a fee for the consultation or charge a higher fee than the current practice in hospitals according to the regulations. Moreover, physicians have to spend relatively more time online compared with the traditional approach [5], because they cannot rely on the health information system to learn the background and medical record of the patients, whom they should fully understand. As a result, the reduced fee [12] and increased time cost lower the willingness of the physicians to offer online consultation.

As the internet hospital is still a very new concept to patients and physicians, there is no sufficient research on the quality and safety of internet hospital and telemedicine care in China. According to a systematic review conducted by McLean et al., there is no difference between the telemedicine for most chronic illnesses and the traditional approaches [6]. However, the safety concern has not been addressed in recent research; and it is uncertain whether the adverse results have not occurred or have not been presented.

6 Opportunities of Internet Hospital in China

The internet hospital and telecommunication technology applications in medical sector have redefined the concept of healthcare delivery. Thanks to the internet hospital, the rural and remote patients' accessibility to as well as the quality of healthcare is significantly improved [9, 15], and the overall healthcare capacity of the rural physicians with the assistance from distant experts is also increased, which helps to provide a more accurate decision in diagnosis, better treatment and follow-up care for rural patients [16]. The close relationship and communication between primary providers and tertiary care providers enable the inexperienced physicians to discover the urgent and severe conditions earlier, consult the opinions of experts in time [17] and ensure that the privilege is given to the referral and inter-hospital transfer for earlier treatment [16]. Meanwhile, the travelling time of specialists is also reduced [18], which, thus, saves both the cost and the lives because of a timely treatment.

Internet hospital overcomes the geographical barriers, makes the easy and low-cost communication between physicians in and outside the country possible, creates opportunities for the collaboration among physicians and supports physicians for distant learning and training [19]. Furthermore, internet hospital connects the healthcare facilities in the area and enables the data to be collected and analyzed, which supports the disaster management, disease management, infectious disease management as well as earlier prevention of epidemic diseases and improves effectively the local communities' capability of health planning and management [6].

With the advancement of telecommunication technologies, the cost of equipment, software and hardware decreases, while the computing speed and internet bandwidths increase, which ensures a better application and experience of internet hospital services. Therefore, patients can be looked after in a better way and managed by remote physicians with improved health outcome.

7 Conclusion

Internet hospital as a new concept to publics, it redefines the healthcare delivery method and prepares to revolutionaries the traditional healthcare industry. With telecommunication technologies, the internet hospital extends affordable and specialist cares to rural and remote locations and improves the health outcome or distant community. Although that the challenges such as quality of care, cost-effectiveness and safety of remote medical treatment are still waiting to be addressed; it is no doubt that internet hospital has a great potential in inter-physician collaboration, distant training and diseases management.

References

1. Tu, J., Wang, C., Wu, S.: The internet hospital: an emerging innovation in China. Lancet Global Health 3(8), e445–e446 (2015)
2. Kelaher, D., Dollery, B.: Health reform in China: an analysis of rural health care delivery. University of New England, School of Economic Studies (2003)
3. Wagstaff, A., Yip, W., Lindelow, M., Hsiao, W.C.: China's health system and its reform: a review of recent studies. Health Econ. 18(Suppl 2), S7–23 (2009)
4. Jennett, P.A., Affleck Hall, L., Hailey, D., et al.: The socio-economic impact of telehealth: a systematic review. J. Telemed. Telecare 9(6), 311–320 (2003)
5. Tian, J.: Construction of network hospital of Guangdong Province in the background of "Internet+Medical". China Digital Medicine. 1, 23–25 (2016)
6. McLean, S., Sheikh, A., Cresswell, K., et al.: The impact of telehealthcare on the quality and safety of care: a systematic overview. PLoS ONE 8(8), e71238 (2013)
7. Li, Y.: Alibaba Blazes a Trail with Online Health Care Pilot. Caixin Online (2016)
8. The World Bank. Urban population (% of total). http://data.worldbank.org/indicator/SP. URB.TOTL.IN.ZS. Accessed 7 June 2016
9. Ebad, R.: Telemedicine: current and future perspectives. Intl. J. Comput. Sci. 10(6), 242–246 (2013)
10. J-z, T.: Hierarchical medical system based on "Internet+Public Healthcare". China Digital Med. 2, 27–28 (2016)
11. China health statistic yearbook 2013 (2013)
12. Wu, Y.: Internet-based smart healthcare changes Chinese lives. The Telegraph (2016)
13. Wuzhen internet Hospital. https://www.guahao.com/. Accessed 18 June 2016
14. Whitten, P.S., Mair, F.S., Haycox, A., May, C.R., Williams, T.L., Hellmich, S.: Systematic review of cost effectiveness studies of telemedicine interventions. BMJ 324(7351), 1434–1437 (2002)
15. Chanussot-Deprez, C., Contreras-Ruiz, J.: Telemedicine in wound care: a review. Adv. Skin Wound Care 26(2), 78–82 (2013)

16. Froehlich, W., Seitaboth, S., Chanpheaktra, N., Pugatch, D.: Case report: an example of international telemedicine success. J. Telemed. Telecare **15**(4), 208–210 (2009)
17. BenZion, I., Helveston, E.M.: Use of telemedicine to assist ophthalmologists in developing countries for the diagnosis and management of four categories of ophthalmic pathology. Clin. Ophthalmol. **1**(4), 489–495 (2007)
18. Kifle, M., Mbarika, V.W.A., Datta, P.: Telemedicine in sub-Saharan Africa: the case of teleophthalmology and eye care in Ethiopia. J. Am. Soc. Inf. Sci. Technol. **57**(10), 1383–1393 (2006)
19. Kvedar, J., Heinzelmann, P.J., Jacques, G.: Cancer diagnosis and telemedicine: a case study from Cambodia. Ann. Oncol. **17**(Suppl 8), viii37–viii42 (2006)

3D Medical Model Automatic Annotation and Retrieval Using LDA Based on Semantic Features

Xinying Wang[1(✉)], Fangming Gu[2], and Wei Xiao[1]

[1] College of Computer Science and Engineering, Changchun University
of Technology, Changchun, China
wang_xinying1979@163.com
[2] College of Computer Science and Technology,
Jilin University, Changchun, China

Abstract. 3D medical model is widely used in many fields such as surgery and medical scene construction. How to find the target model in a large number of 3D models is an important research topic in the field of 3D model retrieval. Due to the existence of semantic gap, the semantic-based method is the current research focus of 3D model retrieval. In this paper, we proposed a semantic-based LDA for automatic 3D medical model annotation and retrieval method. Firstly, we construct semantic features of 3D medical model according to relevance feedback and a small amount of artificial annotation. Then we use the LDA method based on semantic features to obtain latent topic distribution of 3D medical model. Finally, the topic distribution results are applied to automatic annotation of 3D model. Experimental results show that compared with the conventional method of content-based 3D model retrieval, the method can improve the accuracy of 3D medical model automatic annotation and retrieval.

Keywords: Relevance feedback · Unified relationship matrix · Latent Dirichlet Allocation · 3D medical model annotation · 3D medical model retrieval

1 Introduction

A large number of 3D models are produced and widely spread, prompting massive 3D model data requires an efficient retrieval tools to manage and access. The development of 3D model retrieval technology has brought the development opportunity for medical career. Figure 1 is the relationship between 3D model information retrieval and 3D medical model retrieval. Most of the existing content-based retrieval technology is mostly based on the low-level physical features of non-semantic. How to cross the semantic gap between low-level features and high-level semantic concepts, and using the semantic concept to manage and access the 3D model data, has become a hot research topic in the field of multimedia. Among them, the semantic annotation is an important part of overcoming the problem of "semantic gap" and is subject to a long-term focus of research. The traditional manual annotation method has some problem such as low efficiency and consistency of semantic annotation is difficult to ensure, the manual annotation of database technology is difficult to meet practical

© Springer International Publishing AG 2016
X. Yin et al. (Eds.): HIS 2016, LNCS 10038, pp. 91–101, 2016.
DOI: 10.1007/978-3-319-48335-1_10

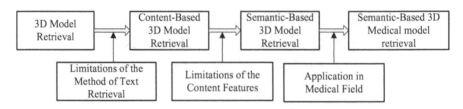

Fig. 1. The relationship between 3D model retrieval and semantic-based medical model retrieval

requirements of large-scale 3D model data. In recent years, automatic annotation of multimedia has gradually become a hot research [1]. High-level semantic classification information can effectively improve the annotation and retrieval efficiency of 3D model.

In the field of text processing, usually using LDA (Latent Dirichlet Allocation) method [2] to classification, this method can discover the hidden semantic structure in document collections. In recent years, LDA method has been widely used in the field of graphics and image processing. For example [3] proposed a method of LDA with saliency information and applied it on aurora image classification. Paper [4] proposed a method based on PCA image reconstruction and LDA for face recognition. Therefore, we consider using the LDA model to solve the problem of 3D model automatic semantic annotation and retrieval. Firstly, we construct semantic features of 3D medical model according to relevance feedback and a small amount of artificial annotation. Then we use the LDA method based on semantic features to obtain latent topic distribution of 3D medical model. Finally, the topic distribution results are applied to automatic annotation of 3D medical model. Experimental results show that compared with the conventional method of content-based 3D model retrieval, the method can improve the accuracy of 3D medical model automatic annotation and retrieval.

2   3D Medical Model Semantic Features

3D model has many semantic features, such as: artificial classification, semantic annotation and so on. In medical field, some 3D models that semantic relationships are closely connected with each other can form a theme, such as "Dental" topic models are shown in Fig. 2.

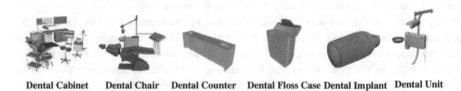

Dental Cabinet   Dental Chair   Dental Counter   Dental Floss Case   Dental Implant   Dental Unit

Fig. 2. Dental topic 3D medical models

This paper mainly uses the user's relevance feedback and a small amount of semantic annotation information to generate the semantic features of 3D medical model, the specific system structure is as follows:

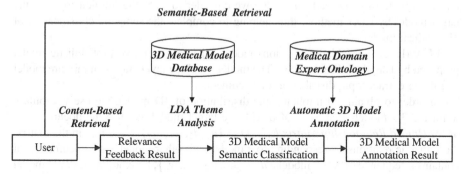

Fig. 3. System structure

In the content-based 3D model retrieval, user's relevance feedback can create an $m \times n$ matrix D, the columns of D are n 3D models in the database and the rows of D are m feedback logs.

D_{ij}, the elements of the matrix D can be defined as:

$$D_{ij} = \begin{cases} 1, & \text{if 3D model } m_j \text{ was marked positive in log } l_i \\ 0, & \text{otherwise} \end{cases}$$

l_i is the i-th line feedback log. D is a sparse matrix, we can accumulate the feedback information of the same target, which can get a $m \times m$ feedback correlation matrix, the matrix can be described a *Unified Relationship Matrix* (*URM*) L_{urm} [6]. L_{urmij}, the element of L_{urm} represents the semantic association strength of 3D model i and 3D model j.

$$L_{urm} = \begin{vmatrix} \lambda_{11}L_{11} & \lambda_{12}L_{12} & \cdots & \lambda_{1N}L_{1N} \\ \lambda_{21}L_{21} & \lambda_{12}L_{22} & \cdots & \lambda_{2N}L_{2N} \\ \vdots & \vdots & \ddots & \vdots \\ \lambda_{N1}L_{N1} & \lambda_{N2}L_{N2} & \cdots & \lambda_{NN}L_{NN} \end{vmatrix} \tag{1}$$

where λ_{ij} is the linear scale weighted coefficient, which can be used to ensure that all kinds of heterogeneous relationships can be compared after linear transformation. In this paper λ_{ij} is 1 and L_{ij} is D_{ij}.

3 Topic Classification of 3D Medical Model Semantic Features

According to the *Unified Relationship Matrix* L_{urm} which structured by semantic feature information of 3D medical model, we consider to infer the implicit topic of the target model by LDA method, thus helping to complete the semantic classification of 3D medical models.

LDA (Latent Dirichlet Allocation) model [2] is a generative probabilistic model proposed by David M. Blei in 2003. The model is a three layer Bayesian mixture model and it can extract topic distribution of document.

In order to obtain the implicit topic distribution of 3D model, we use vocabulary w for the 3D models that associated with the target model and use the document set M for *Unified Relationship Matrix* L_{urm}, $D = \{d_1, d_2, \ldots, d_M\}$. Each row in the matrix, the semantic relations corresponding to a model with other models as a document d, it contains a sequence of N 3D models. $d = \{w_1, w_2, \ldots, w_n\}$, here, w_n is the N 3D model in the sequence.

In *Unified Relationship Matrix* L_{urm}, the matrix elements are represented as discrete digital which is expressed as semantic association strength between two 3D models. In order to be converted into the words in text processing, we use D_{ij} the value of correlation strength to replace with n semantic related 3D model identification directly, then the 3D model identification can be expressed as a vocabulary w in text processing document d.

The method of topic classification of semantic features is as follows:

Suppose there are k topics, the probability of the i-th 3D model w_i in the semantic relationship d can be expressed as follows:

$$P(w_i) = \sum_{j=1}^{T} P(w_i|z_i = j)P(z_i = j) \tag{2}$$

Here, z_i is a potential variable that indicates the i-th 3D model w_i come from the topic, $P(w_i|z_i = j)$ is the probability that model w_i belongs to the topic j, $P(z_i = j)$ is the probability that relationship d belongs to topic j. $\varphi_{w_i}^j = P(w_i|z_i = j)$ represents the multinomial distribution of w 3D models of the j-th topic in the context model, here w is the unique association model of W. $\theta_j^d = P(z_i = j)$ is multinomial distribution of relationship d and T implies topics. Then, the probability d "happen" model w is as follows:

$$P(w|d) = \sum_{j=1}^{T} \varphi_w^j \cdot \theta_j^d \tag{3}$$

Using the expectation maximization algorithm for maximum likelihood function:

$$l(\alpha, \beta) = \sum_{i=1}^{M} \log p(d_i|\alpha, \beta) \tag{4}$$

We need the maximum likelihood estimator α and β, to estimate the parameter values of α and β, so as to determine the LDA model. The conditional probability distribution of associated relationship d is:

$$P(d|\alpha, \beta) = \frac{\Gamma(\sum_i \alpha_i)}{\prod_i \Gamma(\alpha_i)} \int (\prod_{i=1}^{k} \theta_i^{\alpha_i - 1})(\sum_{n=1}^{N} \sum_{i=1}^{k} \prod_{j=1}^{V} (\theta_i \beta_{ij})^{w_n^j}) d\theta \qquad (5)$$

In order to solve θ and β, in LDA model, usually use Gibbs sampling [7] to approximate reasoning algorithm to obtain parameter values to be estimated.

After getting the topic probability of each 3D model, we can divide the 3D model according to the highest probability of the topic it is assigned to. The topic classification results can be used as the results of unsupervised semantic classification of 3D model.

4 3D Medical Model Automatic Annotation

After semantic topic classification, we can get k semantic topics. Suppose that M is the set of 3D medical models in 3D model library and A is the set of 3D models whose semantic information are known, $A \subset M$; if m_i is the 3D medical model in topic T_p, then $\forall m_i \notin A$ and $m_i \in T_p$. The semantic information of m_i can be inferred by the manual annotation of other 3D models in T_p. The detailed strategy states as follows:

(1) If there are some annotated 3D medical models in topic classification T_p and $B_p = (T_p \cap A) \neq \Phi$, $\forall m_i \notin A$ and $m_i \in T_p$, we can sort the 3D models in B_p according to the L_{ij} in L_{urm} descending and then take the largest n different keywords as the semantic annotation of m_i. The basic process, see Fig. 4.

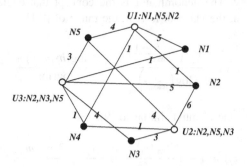

Fig. 4. Strategy 1: annotation method of the unknown 3D models U1, U2 and U3

For example, in Fig. 4, the unlabeled model $U2$ can be annotated with the label of the nearest nodes $N2$, $N5$, and $N3$.

(2) If there are no annotated models in the semantic topic classification T_p, That is to say the set $B_p = (C_p \cap A) \neq \Phi$, then we can look for 3 topic classifications which is the most similar to T_p and has annotated models, thus we can annotate the unknown models according to the method of strategy 1.

Of course, strategy 2 has some defects. Because of the approximate annotation, the annotation accuracy is low (Figs. 4 and 5).

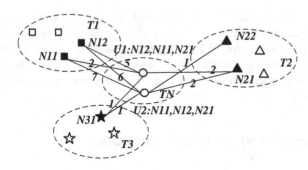

Fig. 5. Strategy 2: annotation method of the unknown 3D models U1 and U2

5 3D Medical Model Semantic Retrieval

The system can calculate the similarity in semantic between keyword W and annotation word S_i according to their semantic relationship in WordNet [8] or medical domain expert ontology. The results of the maximum similarity will be returned to the user.

For a word c of W or S, firstly compute its information content ic using its number of hyponyms with Formula (6). Where the function *hypo* returns the number of hyponyms of a given word and max_{wn} is set to the maximum number of concepts that exist in the taxonomy. The denominator is the concept that contains the maximum amount of information, the value of ic is in the range of [0,1].

$$ic_{wn}(c) = \frac{\log\left(\frac{hypo(c)+1}{max_{wn}}\right)}{\log\left(\frac{1}{max_{wn}}\right)} = 1 - \frac{\log(hypo(c)+1)}{\log(max_{wn})} \tag{6}$$

Then, we propose the formula similar to [9]:

$$sim_{jcn}(c_i, c_j) = 1 - \left(\frac{ic_{wn}(c_i) + ic_{wn}(c_j) - 2 \times sim_{res'}(c_i, c_j)}{2}\right) \tag{7}$$

We can get sim_{res} from the formula below:

$$sim_{res}(c_i, c_j) = \max_{c \in S(c_i, c_j)} ic_{res}(c), c_i \in W, c_j \in S \tag{8}$$

6 Experiment

In experiment, we use 278 3D medical models in PSB [5] and 90 medical 3D models from internet as experiment data. The classification and number of the medical models in PSB is: Skeleton(5), human(100), human_arms_out(41), walking(8), brain(7), face (33), hand(17), head(32), torso(4), skull(6), eyeglasses(7), microscope(5), monitor(13). The classification of the other 90 3D medical model is: Hospital_bed(6), BoneSaw(4), forceps(4), foreceps(4), UtilityCart(7), Walker(6), monitor(5), MedEquip(8), injection (4), others(42). We use the method of depth-buffer [10] to extract the features of 3D model (438 dimensions).

6.1 Annotation Experiment

We use relevance feedback and artificial semantic annotation (<5 %) to get the semantic information of 3D medical model. Then we use them to construct the *Unified Relationship Matrix (URM)* L_{urm}. In the process of relevance feedback, we use the method of content-based 3D model retrieval on the experiment dataset and get 1008 feedback logs from 5 users.

The experiment 3D medical models can be divided into 18 themes based on the LDA method. In order to evaluate the classification performance, we take basic classification of PSB as ground truth, and use the criterions *entropy* and *purity* [11] to evaluate. The definition of *entropy* and *purity* are as follows:

$$Entropy = \sum_{i=1}^{k} \frac{n_i}{N} \left(-\frac{1}{\log q} \sum_{j=1}^{q} \frac{n_i^j}{n_i} \log \frac{n_i^j}{n_i} \right) \tag{9}$$

$$Purity = \sum_{i=1}^{k} \frac{1}{N} \max_j (n_i^j) \tag{10}$$

The bigger Purity and the smaller Entropy value the better classification effect.

Table 1 shows the effect of the proposed method. Obviously, semantic-based LDA performs much better than content-based clustering.

Table 1. Comparison of semantic-based LDA method and content-based feature clustering method

Type	Num. of classifications	Entropy	Purity
Content-based clustering	23	0.398	0.371
LDA topic classification	18	0.260	0.528

We use X-means [12] algorithm to cluster the original shape features and set the number of clusters in the range of 20–25, it is obvious that the classification effect this paper proposed is better than the content-based feature clustering.

Figure 6 lists the results of automatic annotation of some of the topic classification. The annotations marked with underline is the artificial annotation selected randomly, others are automatic annotations.

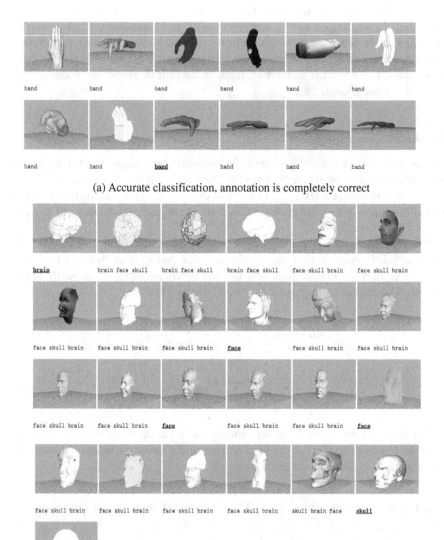

(a) Accurate classification, annotation is completely correct

(b)classification is mess, annotation is substantially correct

Fig. 6. Semantic annotation results

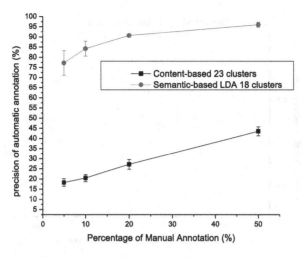

Fig. 7. Average precision curve of automatic annotation

The following figure shows the accuracy of semantic annotation proposed in this paper in different percentages of artificial annotation. Experiment shows that the proposed method is better than the annotation method of content-based feature clustering (Fig. 7).

6.2   Retrieval Experiment

In the retrieval experiment, we compared the proposed method with the method of annotation by content-based features clustering according to the percentage of random artificial annotation. Below is the comparison of two methods of average precision and recall curve (Figs. 8 and 9).

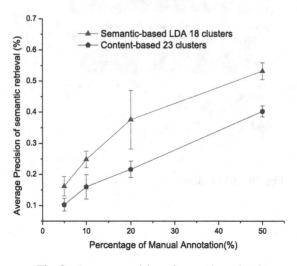

Fig. 8. Average precision of semantic retrieval

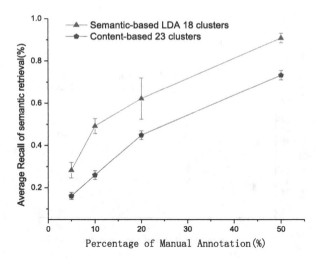

Fig. 9. Average recall of semantic retrieval

It shows that the proposed method is superior to conventional content-based clustering method.

Below is the Screenshot of the 3D medical models semantic retrieval system (Fig. 10).

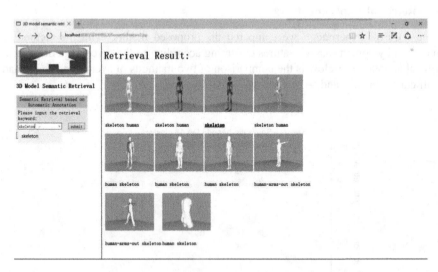

Fig. 10. 3D medical models semantic retrieval system.

7   Conclusion

In this paper, we proposed a method of 3D medical model automatic annotation and retrieval using LDA based on semantic features. Firstly, we construct semantic features of 3D medical model according to relevance feedback and a small amount of artificial annotation. Then we use the LDA method based on semantic features to obtain latent topic distribution of 3D medical model. Finally, the topic distribution results are applied to automatic annotation of 3D medical model. Experimental results show that compared with the conventional method of content-based 3D model retrieval, the method can improve the accuracy of 3D medical model automatic annotation and retrieval.

However, this method also has some shortcomings, if there is no artificial annotation in topic classification, the accuracy of the automatic annotation results will be reduced, thus affecting the efficiency of 3D model retrieval. The improvement of these issues is the focus of our next step.

Acknowledgments. Our work is supported by the National Natural Science Foundation of China under Grant No. 61303132.

References

1. Kumar, A., Dyer, S., Kim, J., et al.: Adapting content-based image retrieval techniques for the semantic annotation of medical images. Comput. Med. Imaging Graph. **49**, 37–45 (2016)
2. Blei, D.M., Ng, A.Y., Jordan, M.I.: Latent Dirichlet allocation. J. Mach. Learn. Res. **3**, 993–1022 (2003)
3. Han, B., Yang, C., Gao, X.B.: Aurora image classification based on LDA combining with saliency information. Ruan Jian Xue Bao/J. Softw. **24**(11), 2758–2766 (2013). (in Chinese)
4. Zhou, C., Wang, L., Zhang, Q., Wei, X.: Face recognition based on PCA image reconstruction and LDA. Optik Int. J. Light Electron Opt. **124**(22), 5599–5603 (2013)
5. Shilane, P., et al.: The Princeton shape benchmark. In: The Shape Modeling International, pp. 388–399 (2004)
6. Xi, W., Fox, E.A., Zhang, B., et al.: SimFusion: measuring similarity using unified relationship matrix. In: SIGIR 2005 Proceedings of the 28th Annual International ACM SIGIR Conference on Research and Development in Information Retrieval, Salvador, Brazil, pp. 130–137, 15–19 August 2005
7. Griffiths, T.L., Steyvers, M.: Finding scientific topics. Proc. Natl. Acad. Sci. **101**(Suppl), 5228–5235 (2004)
8. Felbaum, C.: WordNet: An Electronic Lexical Database. MIT Press, Cambridge (1998)
9. Seco, N., Veale, T., Hayes, J.: An intrinsic information content metric for semantic similarity in WordNet. In: Proceedings of the 16th European Conference on Artificial Intelligence, ECAI 2004, Valencia, Spain (2004)
10. Heczko, M., Keim, D., Saupe, D., Vranic, D.V.: Methods for similarity search on 3D databases. German, Datenbank-Spektrum **2**(2), 54–63 (2002)
11. Zhao, Y., Karypis, G.: Criterion functions for document clustering: experiment and analysis. Technical report, University of Minnesota, 01-40 (2001)
12. Pelleg, D., Moore, A.: X-means: extending k-means with efficient estimation of the number of clusters. In: Proceedings of the 17th International Conference on Machine Learning, ICML 2000, pp. 89–97. Morgan Kaufmann, Palo Alto (2000)

Edge-aware Local Laplacian Filters
for Medical X-Ray Image Enhancement

Jingjing He[1,2(✉)], Mingmin Chen[1,2], and Zhicheng Li[1,2]

[1] Shenzhen Institutes of Advanced Technology, Chinese Academy of Sciences,
Shenzhen, China
hjingjing123@126.com
[2] School of Information Engineering, Wuhan University of Technology,
Wuhan, China

Abstract. This paper proposed a method of edge-aware image processing using standard Laplacian pyramid for medical X-ray image enhancement. It combines edge-aware image processing with multi-scale medical image enhancement algorithm. In particular, after the pyramid decomposition, the large scale edges from small scale detail images are differentiated with a threshold on pixel values. Based on this, a set of image filters are used to achieve edge-preserving smoothing and detail enhancement. The result suggests that our approach enhances the details of the X-ray image by contrast enhancing and edge detail preservation.

Keywords: Edge-aware image processing · Multi-scale enhancement · Laplacian pyramid

1 Introduction

In recent time, Laplacian pyramids were been used to analyze medical images at multiple scales for detail enhancement. This popular method gains ground in image processing until present. For instance, Sun described an improved multi-scale medical image enhancement algorithm. The original Direct Digit Radiography (DR) images can be decomposed into different scales and frequencies of band-pass image sequences by Gaussian and Laplacian pyramid model [1]. For high frequency part of Laplacian pyramid, using multi-scale image enhancement algorithm to enhance details. For the low frequency, we adjust brightness, which can improve contrast of the medical images. Nevertheless, this is not good in edge preserving because some organs and tissues become obscured.

In an attempt to solve this problem, there are some methods about edge-aware image process. In particular, the least-squares scheme [2], the wavelet bases method [3], tone-mapping scheme [4]. However, these decomposition methods are based on filtering thereby enhancing big edges, at the same time small edges being weakened.

This paper was supported by the National 863 Program (2015AA020933) and National Natural Science Foundation of China (61571432, 81571803).

X. Yin et al. (Eds.): HIS 2016, LNCS 10038, pp. 102–108, 2016.
DOI: 10.1007/978-3-319-48335-1_11

Therefore they may cause edge distortion, and gradient inversion (missing details) particularly when applying tone mapping in decomposition.

In order to enhance edges, Fattal adopted gradient-domain method [5]. However, it reconstructs the final image by Poisson equation, not Laplacian pyramid. This cannot combine with classical approaches based on multi-scale image decomposition for details enhancement. Paris presented edge-aware processing using standard Laplacian pyramid [6], but the method aimed at high dynamic images enhancement, not applicable in enhancement of medical images.

In this paper, we propose the approach which combines edge-aware image processing with multi-scale medical image enhancement algorithm. The main contribution of our work is to make up for deficiency (fuzzy edge image) in multi-scale algorithm. In order to solve the problem, we achieved edge-aware image processing through simple point-wise manipulation of Laplacian pyramid. This process is not difficult, but it can retain the edge effectively.

2   Method

Our method is realized by the improved Laplacian pyramid operator. The general process is as shown in Fig. 1. Overview of the basic idea of our approach. After the Gaussian pyramid and Laplacian pyramid of input image are produced, we enhance Laplacian pyramid by multi-scale image enhancement, then based on Gaussian pyramid, we remap the enhanced Laplacian pyramid, and finally we collapse it to give the result.

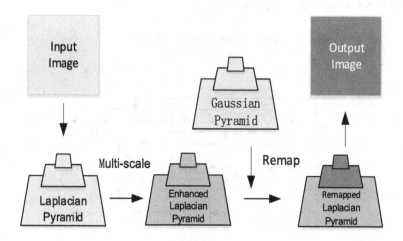

Fig. 1. The general idea of our method

2.1   Laplacian Pyramid

Image pyramid is basis of our approach. It is produced by image decomposition. We make a simple description of its construction. The decomposition process is depicted in

Fig. 2. Given an original image *I*, it is filtered by means of a low pass filter *LP* and subsampled by a factor of two, repeat the process until the top level of pyramid has only a few pixels, then its Gaussian pyramid $\{G_l\}$ are produced. In this Gaussian pyramid, the bottom-most level G_0 is the original image *I*, G_{l+1} is a low-pass version of G_l with half the width and height. The Laplacian pyramid $\{L_l\}$ is constructed on the basis of Gaussian pyramid, first, G_l is inserted a column of zero values every other column, and a row of zero values every other row respectively, then the size of $G_{l(up)}$ is same with G_{l-1}, next, it is filtered by a low-pass filter, $L_{l-1} = G_{l-1} - G_l$, the top level of Gaussian pyramid G_l is L_l, finally, the same process is repeated on the other level of Gaussian pyramid.

2.2 Multi-scale Image Enhancement

The multi-scale image enhancement is based on the decomposition of multiple scales, through the adjustment and reconstruction of image information, to achieve the purpose of image enhancement.

In this paper, we divide Laplacian Pyramid into high frequency and low frequency parts, and deal with them with different algorithms. High frequency images involve more details than low frequency ones and it is clear that an infinite variety of mono-tonically increasing odd mapping functions can be found that will enhance subtle details. The main requirement is that the slope of mapping function is steeper in the region of argument values that correspond to small detail image pixel values or coefficient values than it is in the region of large detail pixel or coefficient values. Therefore, we define a mapping function:

$$g(i) = -m*(-\tfrac{i}{m})^q \quad if\, i < 0 \tag{1}$$

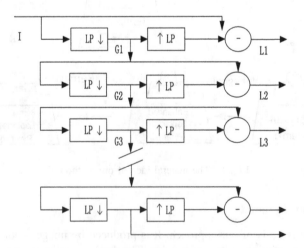

Fig. 2. The generation of Laplacian pyramid

$$g(i) = m*(\frac{i}{m})^q \quad if\, i > 0 \tag{2}$$

Where q is chosen within the interval $0 < q < 1$, preferably within the interval $0.5 < q < 0.9$. m is the maximum of all pixel value in this image.

For low frequency image, its luminance is relatively low, so our method uses a coefficient T to adjust:

$$T = 1 - (-0.2 * \log\frac{|i|}{L_{max}})^p \tag{3}$$

$$f(i) = i*T \tag{4}$$

Typically $0 < p < 1$, it does not work on low frequency images when $p > 1$.

2.3   Edge-aware Laplacian Filter

This processing is realized through the remapping of Laplacian pyramid. This remapping function depends on the image value from the Gaussian pyramid $g_0 = G_0(x_0, y_0)$ and the user parameter σ which is used to distinguish edges from details. For each Gaussian pyramid G_0, there is a corresponding Laplacian pyramid L_0, they are the same size. Based on the g_0, we remap the Laplacian pyramid L_0 using a point-wise function. This process is repeated for each pixel until the output pyramid is produced. As above, the remapping function is related with σ, if $|i - g_0| < \sigma$, it should be processed as detail not edge. We differentiate their treatment by defining two functions h_d and h_e.

$$h_d(i) = g_0 + sign(i - g_0) * \sigma * (\frac{|i-g_0|}{\sigma})^\alpha \quad |i - g_0| < \sigma \tag{5}$$

$$h_e(i) = g_0 + sign(i - g_0) * \beta * (|i - g_0| - \sigma) \quad |i - g_0| > \sigma \tag{6}$$

Where $\alpha > 0$ and $\beta > 0$ is user defined parameter. If $0 < \alpha < 1$, details are enhanced, and if $0 < \beta < 1$, edges are compressed. Furthermore, to avoid the creation of spurious discontinuities, we constrain and to be continuous by requiring that $h_d(g_0 \pm \sigma) = h_e(g_0 \pm \sigma)$.

3   Result

We now demonstrate how to realize practical medical image processing applications using our approach. We processed X-ray image of chest, head and neck, and compared with Sun's multi-scale medical image enhancement algorithm. The result is as shown in Fig. 3. To a certain extent, multi-scale image enhancement method enhances the image details. Compared with original image, the contrast of images is improved.However, the edge of images is not preserved very well. Our method is to process the edges of the image, meanwhile our input image also have an enhancement on the details.

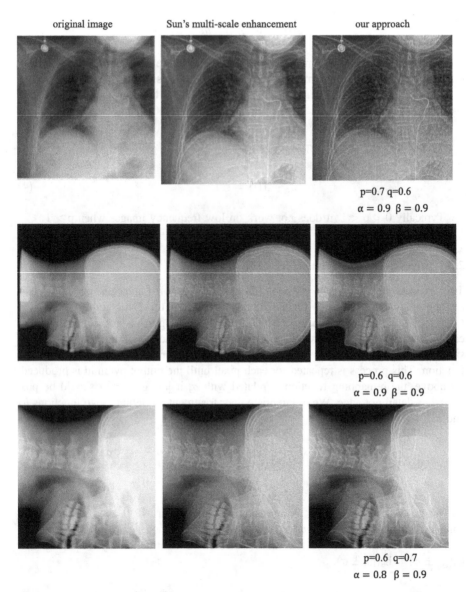

| original image | Sun's multi-scale enhancement | our approach |

p=0.7 q=0.6
α = 0.9 β = 0.9

p=0.6 q=0.6
α = 0.9 β = 0.9

p=0.6 q=0.7
α = 0.8 β = 0.9

Fig. 3. Comparing with multi-scale enhancement, our method enhances the edge and does not smooth the detail at the same time

It can be clearly seen that the spine part of the first group images becomes more prominent, and the outer profile of the head is very clear in the second group images. In the final group images, the neck is enhanced obviously after being processed with our method, and producing no halos. Additionally, processing only two high frequency level, on one hand, it ensures efficient computation, on the other hand, if we process all level of Laplacian pyramid, the result will distort because of processing excessively.

Table 1. Comparison of PSNR of experiment result

Image	Traditional multi-scale enhancement	Our approach
Chest	29.062	34.115
Head	42.124	44.628
Neck	27.205	28.753

Table 1 lists PSNR of experimental results in Fig. 3. The value of PSNR is bigger, the level of image distortion is smaller. From the following table, we can see that compared with the traditional multi-scale enhancement algorithm, our approach can achieve high-quality images.

4 Conclusion

A method of edge-aware local Laplacian filters for medical X-Ray image enhancement is presented in this paper, which combines edge-aware image processing with multi-scale medical image enhancement algorithm. In this way, we apply edge-aware algorithm to medical image processing, it can make up for shortcomings of multi-scale enhancement, which can make image get a better edge preservation as well as enhance the details. In addition, our approach is relatively simple; even so, the result of this method shows it can produce a high-quality result through two complementary algorithms.

References

1. Sun, X.: MultiScale medical image enhancement algorithm. Central South University Of Forestry and Technology (2014, in Chinese) (孙小景. 多尺度医学图像增强算法研究[D]. 中南林业科技大学, 2014)
2. Farbman, Z., Fattal, R., Lischinski, D., Szeliski, R.: Edge-preserving decompositions for multi-scale tone and detail manipulation. ACM Trans. Graph. 27(3), 67:1– 67:10 (2008)
3. Fattal, R.: Edge-avoiding wavelets and their applications. ACM Trans. Graph. 28(3), 22 (2009)
4. Li, Y.Z., Sharan, L., Adelson, E.H.: Compressing and companding high dynamic range images with subband architectures. ACM Trans. Graph. 24(3), 836–844 (2005)
5. Fattal, R., Lischinski, D., Werman, M.: Gradient domain high dynamic range compression. ACM Trans. Graph. 21, 249–256 (2002)
6. Paris, S., Hasinoff, S.W., Kautz, J.: Local Laplacian filters: edge—aware image processing with a Laplacian pyramid. ACM Trans. Graph. 30(4), 68 (2011)
7. Fattal, R., Agrawala, M., Rusinkiewicz, S.: Multiscale shape and detail enhancement from multi—light image collections.ACM Trans. Graph. 26(3), 51 (2007)
8. Lu, J., Healy, D.M., Weaver, J.B.: Contrast enhancement of medical images using multiscale edge representation. Proc. SPIE Intl. Soc. Optical Eng. 33(7), 2151–2161 (1995)
9. Sabine, D., Martin, S., Rafael, W., et al.: Multiscale contrast enhancement for radiographies: Laplacian Pyramid versus fast wavelet transform. IEEE Trans. Med. Imag. 21(4), 343–353 (2002)

10. Subr, K., Soler, C., Durand, F.: Edge-preserving multiscate image decomposition based on local extrema. ACM Trans. Graph. **28**(5), 147:1–147:9 (2009)
11. Tumblin, J., Turk, G.: LCIS: a boundary hierarchy for detail-preserving contrast reduction. ACM Press/Addison-Wesley Publishing Co (1999)
12. Tomasi, C., Manduchi, R.: Bilateral filtering for gray and color images. In: Sixth International Conference on Computer Vision (IEEE Cat. No. 98CH36271), pp. 839–846 (1998)

An Automated Method for Gender Information Identification from Clinical Trial Texts

Tianyong Hao[1], Boyu Chen[1], and Yingying Qu[2(✉)]

[1] School of Informatics, Guangdong University of Foreign Studies,
Guangzhou, China
haoty@gdufs.edu.cn, joey94666@163.com
[2] Faculty of Built Environment, University of New South Wales,
Sydney, Australia
yingyinqu2@gmail.com

Abstract. Gender is fundamental and essential information for eligibility criteria electronic prescreening aiming for recruiting appropriate target population for human studies. Current commonly applied gender architecture contains the problems of incompleteness and ambiguity particularly on transgender. This study designs a flexible and extensible virtual population gender architecture for enhancing trial recruitment. We also propose an automated method for high accurate transgender identification and validation. The method defines and identifies transgender features from free clinical trial text. After that, we apply a context-based strategy to obtain final gender summary. The experiments are based on clinical trials from ClinicalTrials.gov, and results present that the method achieves a True Positive Rate of 0.917 and a True Negative Rate of 1.0 on the clinical trial text, demonstrating its effectiveness in transgender identification.

Keywords: Gender identification · Clinical trial texts · Patient recruitment

1 Introduction

Well-conducted, adequately powered clinical trials are essential to evidence-based medicine and quality-improvement activities [1]. The success of trials heavily relies on the capacity to identify, recruit, and enroll sufficient appropriate target population within a constrained time frame [2, 3]. Recruitment efforts as a substantial proportion of study resources may cost as much as half of the total time for a clinical trial. Consequently, failing to reach recruitment goals imposes significant burdens on patients and healthcare consumers by delaying the translation of new therapies from the laboratory [3–5].

In the recruitment of appropriate participants for human studies, gender is fundamental and essential information for eligibility criteria electronic prescreening. As addressed by Schroeder and Robb [6], gender is often used to establish harvest regulations and strategies, monitor a population's demographic structure, health, and viability, and provide an understanding of behavioral ecology. It is also an essential

© Springer International Publishing AG 2016
X. Yin et al. (Eds.): HIS 2016, LNCS 10038, pp. 109–118, 2016.
DOI: 10.1007/978-3-319-48335-1_12

factor in patient recruitment for clinical trials. Nearly every clinical trial eligibility section specifies the patient gender as a key factor [7, 8]. Moreover, gender is widely used for clinical data retrieval, e.g., the advanced search on clinicaltrials.gov [9]. A recent NIH research project also listed gender as a core element, achieved from international experts in demographics domains [10].

However, current commonly applied gender architecture contains the problems of incompleteness and ambiguity. The problems mainly are: (1) Transgender population is not included, leading to failure in the recruitment of clinical trials for certain types of target population, e.g., HIV related trials commonly require transgender participants. (2) Existing clinical trial registration websites, e.g., ClincialTrials.gov, contain "male", "female", and "both" only, causing the wrong gender registration for the trials targeting for transgender population. Particularly, the numbers of both the transgender population and the trials for transgender recruitment are increasing [11]. As reported by Gary [12] as early as 2011, there are 697,529 adults identified as transgender (about 0.3 % of total adult population) in the United States.

Therefore, an urgent need exists to design a virtual gender architecture to provide more complete and precise population gender types to advance clinical studies and improve target population recruitment. To that end, we design a new architecture of population gender containing both the existing gender types and newly defined transgender types. We further develop an automated transgender identification method through the steps of gender mention identification, context-based feature verification, and gender summarization. Based on the 148,398 clinical trials from ClinicalTrials.gov, our method achieves the performance as a True Positive Rate (sensitivity) of 0.917 and a True Negative Rate (specificity) of 1.0, indicating the effectiveness of the method.

The paper is organized as follows: In Sect. 2, a new gender architecture is introduced. The automated transgender identification method with three steps is presented in Sect. 3. The experiments, results and discussions are presented in Sect. 4, while Sect. 5 summarizes the work.

2 A Virtual Gender Architecture

As a well-recognized official website developed by the National Institute of Health (NIH), Clinicaltrials.gov [9] has been widely accepted by providing a large amount of clinical trial summaries for hospitals, patients, and researchers. As an important criterion, gender is a necessary item in every clinical trial on the website.

However, we manually investigated a number of trials and identified certain problems, which are summarized and categorized into four types: (1) incomplete gender mentions; (2) lack of transgender type; (3) gender type conflict; (4) couple rather than both. Here, we mainly describe the first two problems as this study principally focuses on the transgender issue.

Type 1: incomplete gender mentions
This type of trial requires gender but lacks gender mentions appearing in the criteria text. Taking trial NCT01227343 as an example, it claims "Women ages 18–50 will be eligible for this study..." in Inclusion Criteria section. However, from "Study

Population: Women and men from the greater Philadelphia and surrounding areas who are ages 18–50 will be considered for enrollment into this study" and "Genders Eligible for Study: Both", the criteria should include both male and female, but there is "male" mention missing in the text.

Type 2: lack of transgender type

This kind of problem requires a certain type of transgender population. However, existing clinical trial registration websites, e.g., ClincialTrials.gov, contain "male", "female", and "both" only, causing the difficulty in trial registration. Therefore, wrong gender submissions occur frequently in this type of clinical trial. Taking the clinical trial NCT00435513 as an example, the eligible participants are transgender population according to Study Population section "*Female-to-male transsexuals and male-to-female transsexuals*". However, the gender is incorrectly registered as "*Both*" as there is no option of the "transgender" in submission. Consequently, due to the lack of transgender population included in Genders Eligible for Study section, the recruitment of certain types of transgender population may fail for the clinical trials.

To solve the problems, we firstly define a new gender architecture, as shown in Fig. 1, and then map the existing genders including "male", "female", and "both" to it. The architecture is an extension of commonly used genders to more gender types, including transgender and biological gender. For example, the gender "Male" is mapped to two gender types, "Biological Male" and "Transgender Male", to add the specification of transgender population. Moreover, we intentionally design the archi-tecture as a virtual way considering its flexibility and extension, i.e., the architecture can be further extended or revised as long as the mapping relations are defined.

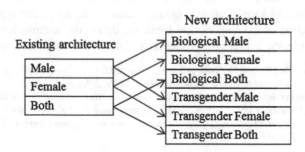

Fig. 1. The definition of a virtual gender architecture and its mapping from existing gender types

Based on the above new gender architecture, we define the relations among the gender types in the architecture to associate all the genders together for relation deduction. As shown in Table 1, there are four types of relations defined including implication relation, reverse relation, constrained equivalence relation, and Topological relation. For example, "*Transgender Male* is equivalent to *Not Transgender Female* in the condition *Transgender*" is a constrained equivalence relation.

Table 1. The definition of gender relations in the architecture

Relation type	Description	Example
Implication relation	x has an implication of y	x = Transgender Female y = Biological Male
Reverse relation	x is NOT y	x = Transgender Male y = Not Transgender Male
Constrained equivalence relation	x is equivalent to y in the condition z	x = Transgender Male y = Not Transgender Female z = Transgender
Expansion relation	y is the expansion of x	x = Transgender Female y = Transgender Both

3   The Method

We therefore propose an automated method for identifying transgender information from free text clinical trials and map them to the new gender architecture. The method includes three steps: (1) gender mention identification; (2) context-based feature verification; (3) gender summarization.

(1)   Gender mention identification

To identify the summary gender for a given clinical trial text, we firstly need to detect gender mentions, which are further mapped to gender types. As a gender type usually has a list of different mentions, we therefore treat the gender mention detection as a process of feature identification to obtain its corresponding gender type. According to the investigation of existing clinical trials, we define the features for each gender type. For example, the features for gender type 'both' and 'transgender' are as follows:

> **Gender 'Both':** *"m/f"*, *"m&f"*, *"both genders"*, *"two genders"*, *"two-gender"*, *"all genders"*, *"all-gender"*, *"male and female"*, *"male&female"*, *"male & female"*
> **Gender 'Transgender':** *"transgender"*, *"transsexual"*, *"transsexuals"*, *"Transsexualism"*, *"change sex"*, *"changed sex"*, *"sex changed"*, *"change gender"*, *"changed gender"*, *"gender changed"*, *"sr surgery performed"*, *"sr surgery"*, *"sex reassignment surgery"*, *"sex reassignment"*, **MFT**, **FMT**

In the example, gender 'both' contains 10 features while 'transgender' contains 16. Particularly, 'transgender' has two feature sets *MFT* (male-to-female transgender) and *FMT* (female-to-male transgender), e.g., *MFT* contains features including *"mft"*, *"female from male"*, *"male to female"*, *"male-to-female"*, *"men transitioning into women"* etc.

After the definition of gender features, we use regular expressions to detect all the mentions in the clinical trial text including the 'purpose' and 'eligibility criteria' section. The free text is split into a number of sentences. Each sentence is then automatically annotated with gender mentions and their corresponding gender types through a strategy combining regular expressions and rules. For example, "*re.sub(r"(? <!(\w|\d|<|>|))(((" +trans+ "))?(" +Tboth+ ")((" +trans+ "))?)(?!(\w|\d|<|>))"*,

'*<G= '+cates1[1]+' '+cates2[0]+r '>\2</G> '*, *text)*" is a regular expression to process a certain type of gender. Applying them on text "*exhibiting some depressive symptomatology i.e., scoring on the beck depression inventory-1a 10 or above, and male or female including transgender female-to-male and male-to-female.*", we can obtain "*transgender*", "*female-to-male*" and "*male-to-female*" as meta gender mentions.

(2) Context-based feature verification

After the feature detection, all the mentions are identified and annotated. We then use a context-based approach to verify the annotations. Some identified gender mentions are context information and should not be included in the final gender summary. For example, "*male*" in "*Two or more male sexual partners in the year prior to study entry*" (NCT00062634) and "*female*" in "*Male Patients with female sexual partners*" (NCT00231465) do not represent the gender of a target population. Those features should be ignored and removed. Therefore, we develop a list of regular expressions to process and correct the annotations.

In addition, certain mention representations are associated with negation words in the same context, which indicates the semantic change. For example, "*transgendered*" in "*Biologically male (not transgendered)*" (NCT01023620) should be ignored. These annotations thus need to be rectified considering the negation situation. To achieve that, we define a list of negation features as "*no*", "*not*", "*without*", "*except*", "*besides*", "*rather*", and "*neither*". After that, we use defined regular expressions to identify the negation features and verify/filter out the gender mentions in the sentence context.

(3) Gender summarization

All the labeled gender mentions are annotated with gender types. We further map them to meta genders in the new architecture, i.e., '*Biological Male*', '*Biological Female*', '*Transgender Male*' and '*Transgender Female*', for the purpose of gender computation. As '*Both*' contains '*Male*' and '*Female*', we split '*Biological Both*' into '*Biological Male*' and '*Biological Female*', while '*Transgender Both*' is split into '*Transgender Male*' and '*Transgender Female*' as well.

With the meta gender types, we sort them by the number of identified mentions. We then design a strategy using majority rule based on the consideration that a text may have multiple gender types and some of them may be noise. If the number of the mentions of the top 1 gender type is larger than that of the second ranked one times a threshold ($Num_{sec} \times \beta$), the system will use the top 1 gender type as the final type directly. Taking NCT02401867 as an example, the original eligible gender is "Female". The purpose section includes "*Preventive Sexual Health Screening Among Female-to-Male FTM Transgender Adult Patients purpose null Study Population. This study aims to enroll 150 female-to-male FTM individuals, ages 21–64. Participants will be recruited from the existing FTM patient population at Fenway Health, ... the aim is to recruit 40 % racial/ethnic minority FTMs*" and the eligibility criteria section includes "*Assigned a female sex at birth and now self-identifies as a man, trans masculine, trans man, FTM, transgender, genderqueer/non-binary, transsexual, male, and/or another diverse transgender identity or expression. Sexually active in the past 36 months with sexual partners of any gender*". There are a number of mentions about "*Transgender Both*". However, our method identifies "*Transgender Male*" type as 7 times and

"*Transgender Both*" as 1, thus "*Transgender Male*" is returned as gender summary result directly when the threshold is 7. Our method filters out the noise mentions and obtains correct result towards the trial purpose.

If no final gender is identified in the process, the system will merge all the identified meta gender types using the relations defined above and record all the results as final gender summary. For example, "*Transgender Female*" and "*Transgender Male*" is merged into "*Transgender Both*".

4   The Experiments and Results

4.1   Datasets

148,398 clinical trials from clinicaltrials.gov as to 2013/07/20 were extracted as experimental dataset. We used certain keywords, e.g., "transgender", "transsexual", and "transsexualism", to extract transgender related clinical trials as a candidate dataset. Three annotators including one clinician and two clinical researchers manually annotated the candidate dataset independently with marked gender types in the new architecture. All the human annotations were reviewed to analyze their differences. For example, as for the sentence "*Male (or transgender) having sex with men*" (NCT01473472), the annotation by the first annotator was ('*Biological Male*', '*Transgender Female*') but was ('*Biological Male*', '*Transgender Male*') by the second annotator. We calculated the inter-agreement as 67.74 % using Fleiss Kappa. Through the discussion, all the differences were eventually solved and a final gold standard thus was established. The examples of the human annotations are shown as Table 2. 44 clinical trials were eventually identified as transgender. We randomly selected 20 trials among them as a training dataset and the other 24 trials as a testing dataset. To further enlarge the experiment dataset, we randomly extracted 22,000 trials marked as non-transgender and separated them as a training and testing dataset too. Finally, we obtained the training dataset (20 transgender trials + 2,000 non-transgender trials) and testing dataset B (24 transgender trials + 20,000 non-transgender trials).

4.2   Evaluation Metrics

We used true positive, true negative, false positive and false negative rates, which are statistical measures of the performance of a binary classification test, as the evaluation metrics [13]. In our experiments, the clinical trials annotated as transgender by human were the positive and the clinical trials annotated as non-transgender were the negative. The clinical trials (gold standard as transgender) annotated as transgender by our method were marked as true positive (TP) case. The clinical trials (gold standard as non-transgender) annotated as non-transgender were marked as true negative (TN) case. The clinical trials (gold standard as non-transgender) annotated as transgender were marked as false positive (FP) case. The clinical trials (gold standard as transgender) annotated as non-transgender were marked as false negative (FN) case. These were the formulas for calculating the four evaluation metrics: sensitivity as TP rate = $TP/(TP + FN)$, specificity as TN rate = $TN/(TN + FP)$, FP rate = $FP/(TN + FP)$

Table 2. The samples of the gold standard and the annotations from three human annotators

Trial ID	Original	Gold standard	Annotator 1	Annotator 2	Annotator 3
NCT00111501	Both	'Biological Both', 'Transgender Both'	'Biological Both', 'Transgender Both'	'Biological Both', 'Transgender Both'	'Biological Both', 'Transgender Both'
NCT00135148	Female	'Biological Female', 'Transgender Female'	'Biological Female', 'Transgender Female'	'Biological Female', 'Transgender Female'	'Biological Female', 'Transgender Female'
NCT00146146	Female	'Biological Female', 'Transgender Male'	'Transgender Male'	'Biological Female', 'Transgender Male'	'Transgender Male'
NCT00241202	Both	'Biological Both', 'Transgender Both'	'Biological Both', 'Transgender Both'	'Transgender Both'	'Biological Both', 'Transgender Both'
NCT00435513	Both	'Transgender Both'	'Transgender Both'	'Transgender Both'	'Biological Both', 'Transgender Both'
NCT00634218	Both	'Biological Both', 'Transgender Both'	'Biological Both', 'Transgender Both'	'Biological Both', 'Transgender Both'	'Biological Both', 'Transgender Both'
NCT00865566	Male	'Biological Male', 'Transgender Female'	'Biological Male', 'Transgender Female'	'Biological Male', 'Transgender Both'	'Biological Male', 'Transgender Female'
NCT01065220	Both	'Transgender Both'	'Transgender Both'	'Transgender Both'	'Transgender Both'
NCT01072825	Both	'Transgender Both'	'Transgender Both'	'Transgender Both'	'Transgender Both'
NCT01283360	Male	'Biological Male', 'Transgender Female'	'Biological Male', 'Transgender Female'	'Biological Male', 'Transgender Female'	'Biological Male', 'Transgender Female'

and FN rate = $FN/(TP + FN)$. Our purpose was to maximize the TP rate (sensitivity) and TN rate (specificity), while minimizing the FP rate and FN rate.

4.3   Parameter Tuning

We firstly acquired the optimized threshold parameter β described in Sect. 3. The training dataset was processed by our method with the threshold being set from 1 to 10. The system performances, as TP rate, TN rate, FP rate and FN rate, were calculated. As shown in Table 3, the results showed that the TP rate obtained the highest value and the FN rate obtained the lowest when the thresholds were 7 or 8. We reviewed the results comprehensively and identified $\beta = 7$ as the optimized value.

4.4   The Results and Discussions

Using the $\beta = 7$, our method processed the testing dataset with the non-transgender text increasing from 50 to 10000. The TP rate, TN rate, FP rate and FN rates of the different non-transgender data results were calculated. As shown in Fig. 2, the results demonstrated that our method achieved stable performance on all the evaluation metrics. The experiments also demonstrated that our method is stable in processing transgender texts regardless of the increasing number of non-transgender texts.

After that, we applied the method on all the testing dataset containing 20000 non-transgender trials. As there are no similar work and baseline methods available in the transgender identification from free text for comparison, we mainly report our results in the paper. It achieved a True Positive Rate of 0.917, a True Negative Rate of 1.0, a False Positive Rate of 0, and a False Negative Rate of 0.083. This indicated that all the non-transgender trials were correctly identified. All the transgender trials were correctly identified as transgender type, and 91.7 % were correctly annotated compared with human annotations. 8.3 % of transgender cases were incorrectly identified as error cases.

In addition, we analyzed all the error cases by our method and identified the following types:

(1) Context problem. For the text "*Young men who have sex with men (MSM) that obtain medical care from a Gay/Lesbian/Bisexual/Transgender community health clinic*" in NCT01197079, the gender was '*Biological Male*' in gold standard but it processed the attributive clause "*Transgender*" and marked it as '*Transgender Both*'. For the text "*Hemoglobin (Hgb) greater than or equal to 10.5 g/dL for volunteers who were born female, greater than or equal to 13.0 g/dL for volunteers who were born male*" in NCT02716675, our method annotated "*female*" as '*Biological Female*' in the sentence. However, the clinical trial aimed to recruit "*men and transgender (TG) persons*". It showed that the context including irrelevant information could lead to incorrect gender identification.

(2) Semantic problem. For the text "*Healthy biological females, between 18 and 45 years of age*" and "*SR surgery performed*" in NCT00146146, "*SR surgery performed*" was annotated as '*Transgender Both*', which was further merged with '*Biological Female*' as '*Transgender Both*' by our method. However, human annotators treated the two separate sentences together and regarded the semantic of the two sentences as '*Transgender Male*' only. Another example is on the text "*All transsexual women treated according to the Standards of Care of the World Professional Association of*

Table 3. The performance using different threshold values

β	TP rate	TN rate	FP rate	FN rate
1	0.2	1.0	0.0	0.8
2	0.65	1.0	0.0	0.35
3	0.7	0.995	0.005	0.3
4	0.85	0.995	0.005	0.15
5	0.85	0.995	0.005	0.15
6	0.85	0.995	0.005	0.15
7	0.9	0.995	0.005	0.1
8	0.9	0.995	0.005	0.1
9	0.85	0.995	0.005	0.15
10	0.85	0.995	0.005	0.15

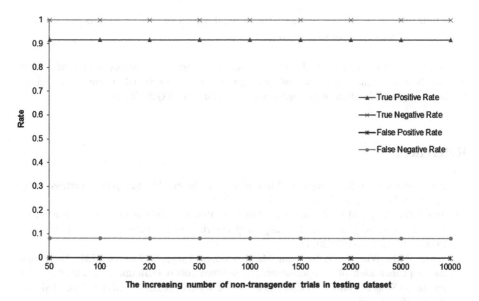

Fig. 2. The performance with the increasing number of non-transgender trials in the testing dataset

Transgender Health (WPATH)" and *"Participants underwent the sex reassignment surgery (SRS)..."* in NCT01708148. The method annotated *"sex reassignment surgery"* as *'Transgender Both'* but human annotators considered the semantics together and annotated it as *'Transgender Female'*. The complexity of semantics thus was another issue affecting the performance of transgender identification.

For the two error types, we plan to introduce syntactic analysis to identify gender mention modifiers and clauses so as to identify the context of gender mentions. After that, we will try to merge the possible mentions together upon their semantic meaning and predefined relations.

As the accumulated clinical trials contain fixed gender information, our method needs to process the trials only once and records identified gender results for further reuse. Therefore, there is only minor over-heading problem on the system performance in processing all clinical trials.

5 Summary

Gender is fundamental and essential information for eligibility criteria prescreening for recruiting appropriate participants for human studies. This research conducted an investigation of eligibility criteria texts and proposed a new virtual gender architecture by incorporating transgender populations and defined the mapping relations between existing genders to the architecture. We further proposed an automated method for high accurate gender identification and validation. The method proceeded clinical texts with gender mention identification, context-based feature verification, and gender summarization steps. Experiments on the clinical trials from ClincialTrials.gov demonstrated the effectiveness of the proposed method.

Acknowledgements. The work described in this paper was substantially supported by the National Natural Science Foundation of China (grant No. 61403088) and the Innovative School Project in Higher Education of Guangdong, China (grant No. YQ2015062).

References

1. Fernández-Arroyo, S., Camps, J., Menendez, J.A., Joven, J.: Managing hypertension by polyphenols. Planta Med. **81**(08), 624–629 (2015)
2. Tua, S.W., Pelega, M.B., Carinic, S., Bobakc, M., Rossd, J., Rubine, D., Simc, I.: A practical method for transforming free-text eligibility criteria into computable criteria. J. Biomed. Inform. **44**(2), 239–250 (2011)
3. Jeffrey, M.F., William, G., Jonathan, M., Howard, S., Tanya, B., Monica, M.H.: The design and implementation of an open-source, data-driven cohort recruitment system: the Duke Integrated Subject Cohort and Enrollment Research Network (DISCERN). J. Am. Med. Inf. Assoc. **19**(e1), e68–e75 (2012)
4. Weng, C., Wu, X., Luo, Z., Boland, M.R., Theodoratos, D., Johnson, S.B.: EliXR: an approach to eligibility criteria extraction and representation. J. Am. Med. Inform. Assoc. **18** (Suppl 1), i116–i124 (2011)
5. Hao, T., Rusanov, A., Boland, M.R., Weng, C.: Clustering clinical trials with similar eligibility criteria features. J. Biomed. Inform. **52**, 112–120 (2014)
6. Schroeder, M.A., Robb, L.A.: Criteria for gender and age. Techniques for wildlife investigations and management, pp. 303–338 (2005)
7. Weng, C., Tu, S.W., Sim, I., Richesson, R.: Formal representation of eligibility criteria: a literature review. J. Biomed. Inform. **43**(3), 451–467 (2010)
8. Lonsdale, D., Tustison, C., Parker, C., Embley, D.W.: Formulating queries for assessing clinical trial eligibility. In: Kop, C., Fliedl, G., Mayr, H.C., Métais, E. (eds.) NLDB 2006. LNCS, vol. 3999, pp. 82–93. Springer, Heidelberg (2006)
9. Clinicaltrials.gov-A service of the U.S. National Institutes of Health. http://clinicaltrials.gov/ Accessed in 2016
10. Lynch, D.R., Pandolfo, M., Schulz, J.B., Perlman, S., Delatycki, M.B., Payne, R.M., Shaddy, R., Fischbeck, K.H., Farmer, J., Kantor, P., Raman, S.V., Hunegs, L., Odenkirchen, J., Miller, K., Kaufmann, P.: Common data elements for clinical research in friedreich's ataxia. Mov. Disord. **28**(2), 190–195 (2013)
11. Cichocki, M.: HIV risk in the transgender men and women - understanding why transgender people are at increased HIV risk. https://www.verywell.com/hiv-risk-and-the-transgender-population-47883. Accessed in 2016
12. Gates, G.J.: How many people are lesbian, gay, bisexual, and transgender? The Williams Institute, UCLA (2011)
13. Lalkhen, A.G., McCluskey, A.: Clinical tests: sensitivity and specificity. BJA: CEACCP **8**(6), 221–223 (2008)

A Novel Indicator for Cuff-Less Blood Pressure Estimation Based on Photoplethysmography

Hongyang Jiang[1,2], Fen Miao[1], Mengdi Gao[2], Xi Hong[1,3],
Qingyun He[1], He Ma[2], and Ye Li[1(✉)]

[1] Key Laboratory for Health Informatics of the Chinese Academy
of Sciences (HICAS), Shenzhen Institutes of Advanced Technology,
Shenzhen, People's Republic of China
{hy.jiang,fen.miao,xi.hong,qy.he,ye.li}@siat.ac.cn
[2] Sino-Dutch Biomedical and Information Engineering School,
Northeastern University, Shenyang, People's Republic of China
{hongyang1020,neugaomengdi}@126.com,
mahe@bmie.neu.edu.cn
[3] Optical and Electronic Information School, Huazhong University of Science
and Technology, Wuhan, People's Republic of China

Abstract. Cuff-less blood pressure (BP) measurement provides an efficient way to estimate blood pressure and thus prevent cardiovascular disease caused by hypertension. Pulse transit time (PTT) based BP estimation model has attracted much interests but with limited application. The measurement of PTT needs two photoplethysmographic (PPG) sensors or one electrocardiogram (ECG) sensor and one PPG sensor and thus restricted its widespread acceptance. In this study, a novel indicator, Photoplethysmography Acceleration Ratio (PAR), is extracted from the second-order derivative of PPG signal, which is validated as a significant parameter for estimating BP. 120 subjects, aged from 18 to 84, participated in this experiment. The results show that the correlation coefficient between PAR and systolic, diastolic and mean BP are 0.701, 0.331 and 0.629 respectively. Furthermore, the performance of accuracy and precision is good through correlation analysis. Therefore, the proposed PAR is demonstrated to be useful for SB measurement with only one sensor.

Keywords: Cuff-less blood pressure · Photoplethysmography Acceleration Ratio · Correlation analysis

1 Introduction

Blood pressure (BP) is the major risk factor for predicting cardiovascular events [1]. High BP (hypertension) and low BP (hypotension) reflect the abnormal physiological status of people. Hypertension is becoming more prevalent but poorly controlled due to low awareness, even in young people under 40, and thus creates great burdens on the society. Ubiquitous BP measurement is significant to improve hypertension and pre-hypertension patient management by providing continuous BP monitoring.

Currently, cuffs are used for blood pressure measurement. However, blood pressure machine with cuff for inflation is big in size and inconvenient for use, therefore cannot

© Springer International Publishing AG 2016
X. Yin et al. (Eds.): HIS 2016, LNCS 10038, pp. 119–128, 2016.
DOI: 10.1007/978-3-319-48335-1_13

fulfill the requirement of monitoring BP anytime and anywhere. Recent cuff-less blood pressure estimation approach based on Pulse Transit Time (PTT) has been studied in [2–4] and has achieved reasonable accuracy. However, these approaches are not very straightforward as the measurement of PTT needs two photoplethysmographic (PPG) sensors or one electrocardiogram (ECG) sensor and one PPG sensor. Calibration is also needed in such approaches. By taking this situation into consideration, some studies presented blood pressure estimation method with features extracted from just one PPG sensor [5–7]. Satomi et al. [5] took advantage of several points of acceleration pulse wave to estimate blood pressure based only on photoplethysmogram. In his experiment, the age of volunteers were divided into more than 60 and less than 60. Hayato Fukushima et al. [6, 7] constructed blood pressure model with CO (Cardiac Output) and TPR (Total Peripheral Resistance), both of which were measured by Finometer Pro, a product of Finapres Medical Systems Corp. Although those methods obtained good results that are closed to AAMI requirement, some complex measurement steps may limit their application and promotion. Novel indicators for BP should be further studied to improve accuracy and convenience of cuff-less measurement.

In this paper, we propose a novel BP estimation indicator Photoplethysmography Acceleration Ratio (PAR) extracted from one single PPG signal, which is easy to collect. The normalized waveform of PPG and acceleration PPG (APG) are shown as Fig. 1 and the indicator PAR is extracted from APG signals. With the help of PAR, we can reduce the complexity of the BP measurement and enhance the portability of BP measurement products. Significantly, it provides a promising attempt for constructing a more accurate BP estimation model that can be combined with other techniques.

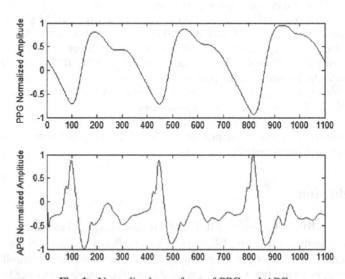

Fig. 1. Normalized waveform of PPG and APG.

2   Method

2.1   Subjects and Experiment Protocol

In this study, a total of 120 subjects were recruited for data collection. An informed consent was obtained from each subject and this experiment was approved by institutional ethics committee. The experimental cohorts consisted of healthy groups and high blood pressure groups where participants were engaged in various occupations.

Three-In-One, a portable physiological signal acquisition system designed by Shenzhen Institute of Advanced Technology (SIAT), was used to collect PPG signals of subjects using the sample frequency of 500 Hz. OMRON HEM-1020 electronic sphygmomanometer was used to measure subjects' blood pressures. The basic data collection procedures contained following steps:

- Subjects rest for 5 min before data collection.
- Subjects sit in upright posture. Blood pressure is measured by OMRON HEM-1020, and denoted as BP_1.
- Subjects keep sitting and PPG signal from middle finger is gathered for 1 min by Three-In-One.
- After finishing PPG signals collection, blood pressure is measured again immediately and denoted as BP_2.

During the data collection, the average blood pressure, symbolized as BP_a, can be calculated by averaging BP_1 and BP_2:

$$BP_a = (BP_1 + BP_2)/2. \tag{1}$$

BP_a can be approximate to the average blood pressure during this 1 min time. Meanwhile, index finger transmittance PPG signals are recorded and saved.

2.2   Data Preprocessing

Through data collection steps described above, 1 min PPG signals sequences gathered from each subject were saved in computer. As Three-In-One equipment is an integrated and portable physiological signal acquisition circuit board, low complexity is one of its features. Because the raw PPG signals were mixed with noises that include low frequency and high frequency signals, a digit band-pass filter program was designed to eliminate those noises. Moreover, a smoothing algorithm was applied to these signals. This study implemented three-time-seven-point smooth processing using following formula:

$$
\begin{aligned}
y_{(i)} = -\,(2x_{(i-3)} + 6x_{(i-2)} + 12x_{(i-1)} + 14x_{(i)} \\
+ 12x_{(i+1)} + 6x_{(i+2)} + 2x_{(i+3)})/21,
\end{aligned} \tag{2}
$$

where input x represented raw PPG signals and output y is smoothed PPG signals.

2.3   Feature Points Selection and Data Filtration

Numerous features based on electrocardiogram (ECG) and PPG have been proposed by many researchers. However, more features do not necessarily mean better results and it is not enough to utilize these features for accurate blood pressure estimation. More concerns should be focused on appropriate and effective features selection. Changes in blood volume produce PPG, i.e. pulse wave. Through second-order differential, APG can be obtained from PPG and is reported as a more practical waveform that has clear features [8]. These feature points and their combination have been also shown to be meaningful by many studies [3, 5, 6, 10, 11]. Furthermore, APG is associated with some symptomatic risk factors such as systolic blood pressure and diastolic blood pressure [9]. Figure 2 shows some feature points of APG.

The waveform between two waves' peak points, contains a large amount of undiscovered useful information. These features including peak and valley points a, b, c, d, e, f that have been proposed and used by previous researches [10, 11]. This study employed a new point g, which is located at the end of the current waveform and is close to peak point a of next wave.

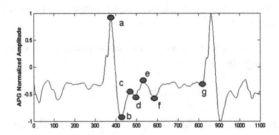

Fig. 2. Features of acceleration PPG signal.

As a matter of fact, the positions of peak or valley points c, d, e, f are difficult to capture because of the influence of environment, postures and measuring equipment, especially when portable measurement equipments are used. In addition, for many subjects some of the four clear points cannot be observed clearly. The error rate of feature extraction is quite high. Hence, this study automatically extracted point d and g instead of the entire set of points, as shown in Fig. 3.

Different ages and physical conditions may create variations in the shapes of points. Furthermore, some waveforms of the subjects have inconspicuous standard points d due to individual difference, so the point d does not always appear as a valley point, as shown in Fig. 4(a). In this situation, this study considered the point with minimum slope between point b and e as the correct point d. This type of point d and standard point d are shown in Fig. 4.

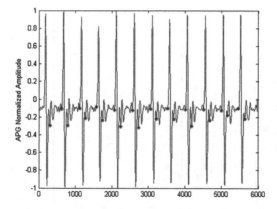

Fig. 3. Extraction of feature point d and g.

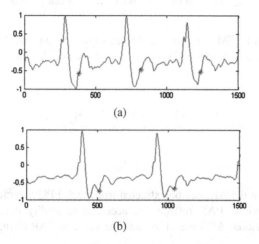

Fig. 4. Two types of point d. (a) Point with minimum slope between point b and e. (b) Standard point as a valley point.

2.4   Proposed Feature

After the feature points d and g are extracted, we can get the section of signal waveform between point d and g. We can truncate this section from the whole signal waveform, as shown in Fig. 5. The waveform contains other undefined feature points that influence the shape of this waveform to a great extent.

In this study, we proposed a novel feature θ, which was an angle calculated from the extracted signal waveform. First, we set point d as the initial point, and point g as the end point of a points sequence $Y = \{y_1, y_2, \ldots, y_n\}$ with a corresponding discrete time sequence $X = \{1, 2, \ldots, n\}$. Second, using these pairs of discrete points, a fitted regression line equation such as (3) was constructed using the least squares fitting method (LSFM). From the gradient of this line the accelerating rate of artery blood flow was

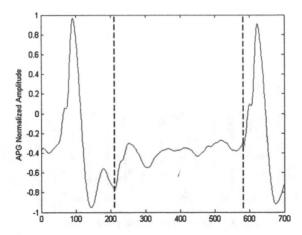

Fig. 5. Segmentation of signal waveform between point d and g.

calculated. Through LSFM, we can calculate this gradient p using the Eq. (4). Finally, using the transformation function (5), we obtained the angle θ, which is shown in Fig. 6.

$$y = p \cdot x + q \tag{3}$$

$$p = \frac{6n\left[2\left(\sum_{i=1}^{n} i \cdot y_i\right) - (n+1)\left(\sum_{i=1}^{n} y_i\right)\right]}{n^2(n^2 - 1)} \tag{4}$$

$$\theta = \arctan(p) \tag{5}$$

The angle θ, that is PAR, can be extracted from each PPG waveform cycle. From a physical point of view, PAR reflects the accelerating ability between point d and g provided by individual APG waveform and the value of PAR changes along with the PPG waveform.

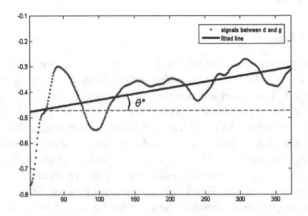

Fig. 6. Linear fit chart between point d and g.

3 Experiment and Result

3.1 Data Description

120 subjects were randomly recruited in this experiment and the age of them ranged from 18 to 84 years old. All of their PPG signals were collected and saved in the computer. The experiment steps are as follows:

- Through observation, 7 distorted signals were abandoned and 113 signals were picked out.
- Based on the feature point d, the signals consisted of two groups. Members of Group A (95 signals) had clear valley point d in their waveforms and members of Group B (18 signals) do not.
- Feature extraction was done on both Group A and Group B separately.
- Data analysis was executed and blood pressure estimation was made using regression method.

Among the subjects, there were 59 males and 54 females. Table 1 shows the age distribution of these subjects. Their SBP is shown in Table 2 and some of the subjects were hypertension patients.

Table 1. Age distribution of subjects

Age (years)	~ 20	$21 \sim 40$	$41 \sim 60$	$61 \sim$
Subjects' number	2	42	32	37

Table 2. SBP distribution of subjects

SBP (mmHg)	$80 \sim 100$	$101 \sim 120$	$121 \sim 140$	$141 \sim$
Subjects' number	7	46	39	21

3.2 Performance of the Proposed Indicator in BP Estimation

Using the indicator PAR, which is proposed to track the BP of subjects, we get equations for systolic blood pressure (SBP), mean artery pressure (MAP) and diastolic blood pressure (DBP) estimation through polynomial regression method. A correlation analysis was first performed between the proposed PAR and SBP, MAP, DBP respectively using Pearson's correlation in SPSS. The results are shown in Table 3. From Table 3 we can see that PAR shows significant correlation with SBP, MAP and DBP ($p < 0.01$), especially with the SBP, where the Pearson correlation coefficient is over 0.7. Thus PAR is a potential indicator of SBP.

Table 3. Pearson correlation analysis

	Pearson correlation	Sig. (2-tailed)	No. of samples
PAR vs. SBP	0.701	.000	113
PAR vs. MAP	0.629	.000	113
PAR vs. DBP	0.331	.003	113

To verify the effectiveness of PAR in estimating BP, univariate linear regression analysis was used for modeling BP. The fitted models and residuals analysis for SBP, MAP and DBP are presented in Figs. 7, 8 and 9 respectively. From the figures we can see that PAR and BP basically conform to a linear model, especially for PAR and SBP. We also evaluate the performance of the fitted model in terms of mean difference (MD) ± standard deviation (SD) and mean absolute difference (MAD) of the estimated BP with the reference blood pressure. The results are presented in Table 4. We can see that even though the mean errors are small, the standard deviations should be further improved to conform to AAMI standard.

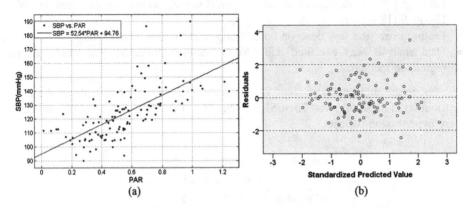

Fig. 7. (a) Linear regression of SBP. (b) Residuals plot of predicted SBP.

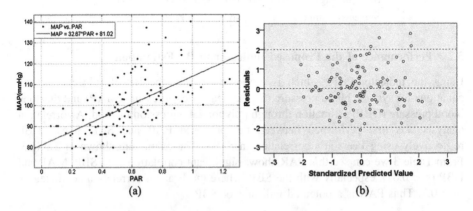

Fig. 8. (a) Linear regression of MAP. (b) Residuals plot of predicted MAP.

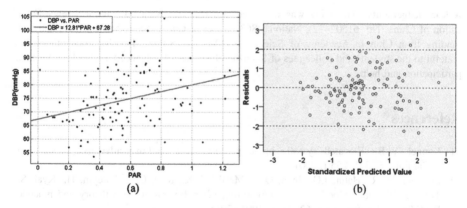

Fig. 9. (a) Linear regression of DBP. (b) Residuals plot of predicted DBP.

Table 4. Accuracy, precision between estimated BP and the reference

	SBP	MAP	DBP
R-square	0.4925	0.3967	0.1098
Adjusted R-square	0.4879	0.3912	0.1018
MD ± SD (mmHg)	$-1.95 \times 10^{-16} \pm 13.81$	$9.34 \times 10^{-17} \pm 10.44$	$7.00 \times 10^{-15} \pm 9.45$
MAD (mmHg)	10.9	8.64	7.59

4   Discussion and Conclusion

As presented in [11], the PPG patterns are distinctive in different population groups. Due to individual differences and physiological status such as activity and nervous, we also found some APG waveforms have no obvious d point or the d point does not appear in the PPG waveform. To solve this problem, this study presented the minimum slope method to locate the probable position of point d. However, the correct results acquired by this method is probabilistic. In the future, an efficient method to handle this kind of signals should be further studied to gain wider acceptance of the proposed model. However, the development of the PAR indicator represents a new research direction for monitoring BP, and may produce ultimate indicators of BP estimation. Besides, the waveforms of PPG and its transformation forms play an important role in BP monitoring, so more significant features should be further discovered and extracted from them, such as latent parameters of PPG [12]. Hence, more accurate BP estimation equation will be further created through statistical methods and machine learning technologies.

In this study, we proposed a novel indicator PAR for cuff-less BP estimation. The experiment on 113 subjects that included hypertensive patients and health people shows that PAR is high correlated with BP. Therefore, with the help of PAR, we may realize portable, generalized and high precision BP measurement in the future by merging more features into the BP-estimation model.

Acknowledgements. This work was supported in part by the National Natural Science Foundation of China (No. 61502472), National 863 project of China (SS2015AA020109) and STS funding from Chinese Academy of Sciences (KFJ-EW-STS-095). Besides, the authors feel grateful to the students and colleagues of Shenzhen Institutes of Advanced Technology for their participation and help.

References

1. Kannel, W.B.: Elevated systolic blood pressure as a cardiovascular risk factor. Am. J. Cardiol. **85**, 251–255 (2000)
2. Mukkamala, R., Hahn, J.O., Inan, O.T., Mestha, L.K., Kim, C.S., Toreyin, H., Kyal, S.: Toward ubiquitous blood pressure monitoring via pulse transit time: theory and practice. IEEE Trans. Biomed. Eng. **62**, 1879–1901 (2015)
3. Kachuee, M., Kiani, M.M., Mohammadzade, H., Shabany, M.: Cuff-less high-accuracy calibration-free blood pressure estimation using pulse transit time. In: IEEE International Symposium on Circuits and Systems, pp. 1006–1009 (2015)
4. Gesche, H., Grosskurth, D., Küchler, G., Patzak, A.: Continuous blood pressure measurement by using the pulse transit time: comparison to a cuff-based method. Eur. J. Appl. Physiol. **112**, 309–315 (2012)
5. Suzuki, S., Oguri, K.: Cuff-less and non-invasive systolic blood pressure estimation for aged class by using a photoplethysmograph. In: 30th IEEE International Conference Engineering on Medicine and Biology Society, Vancouver, British Columbia, Canada, pp. 1327–1330 (2008)
6. Fukushima, H., Kawanaka, H., Bhuiyan, M.S., Oguri, K.: Cuff-less blood pressure estimation using only photoplethysmography based on cardiovascular parameters. In: 35th IEEE International Conference Engineering on Medicine and Biology Society, Osaka, Japan, pp. 2132–2135 (2013)
7. Hodgson, Y., Choate, J.: Continuous and noninvasive recording of cardiovascular parameters with the Finapres finger cuff enhances undergraduate student understanding of physiology. Adv. Physiol. Educ. **36**, 20–26 (2012)
8. Song, S.H., Cho, J.S., Oh, H.S., Lee, J.S., Kim, I.Y.: Estimation of blood pressure using photoplethysmography on the wrist. In: Computers in Cardiology, pp. 741–744 (2009)
9. Takada, H., Washino, K., Harrell, J.S., Iwata, H.: Acceleration plethysmography to evaluate aging effect in cardiovascular system. Using new criteria of four wave patterns. Med. Prog. Technol. **21**, 205–210 (1995)
10. Takazawa, K., Tanaka, N., Fujita, M., Matsuoka, O., Saiki, T., Aikawa, M., Tamura, S., Ibukiyama, C.: Assessment of vasoactive agents and vascular aging by the second derivative of photoplethysmogram waveform. Hypertension **32**, 365–370 (1998)
11. Suzuki, A., Ryu, K.: Feature selection method for estimating systolic blood pressure using the Taguchi method. IEEE Trans. Ind. Inform. **10**, 1077–1085 (2014)
12. Datta, S., Banerjee, R., Choudhury, A.D., Sinha, A., Pal, A.: Blood pressure estimation from photoplethysmogram using latent parameters. In: IEEE International Conference on Communications, Kuala Lumpur, Malaysia, pp. 1–7 (2016)

A Dietary Nutrition Analysis Method Leveraging Big Data Processing and Fuzzy Clustering

Lihui Lei[✉] and Yuan Cai

School of Computer Science, Shaanxi Normal University, Xi'an 710062, China
{leilihui, caiyuan}@snnu.edu.cn

Abstract. Dietary nutrition analysis is important because it can provide scientific guidances for human to keep healthy and administrative departments to make rational decisions. However, the existing dietary nutrition analysis methods need to be improved. On the one hand, the data to be processed should be more accurate. Most methods use a sample taken at a moment time to represent all samples produced during a period of time, which neglects the fact samples may change over time. On the other hand, data analysis should be efficiently and effectively, as the number of samples is rapidly increasing and the types of samples are constantly emerging. This paper introduces a new method. Firstly, samples are preprocessed using a data model obtained by big data processing. Secondly, the fuzzy c-means algorithm is parallelized with Mapreduce for data analysis. The optimization rules are given. Finally, the experiments prove that this method is efficiently and effectively.

Keywords: Dietary nutrition analysis · Fuzzy clustering · Big data · Mapreduce

1 Introduction

Dietary nutrition analysis is very important, because it not only can make individuals know whether their diet is reasonable to keep themselves healthy, but also can make management departments know the overall dietary nutrition status of some groups (e.g., sports teams) to adopt scientific management strategy. Jie jiang et al. [1] used both the statistical methods and the biochemical methods to analyzed the metal elements in human intakes. However, which and how much ingredients are consumed by the residents are estimated based on statistical methods, therefore the dietary metal elements intake of the residents is estimated roughly. The literatures [2] presented the similar methods. ChangLin Yang [3] developed a kind of nutrition analysis software based on a statistical analysis for different professional groups (e.g., pilots, athletes). The literatures [4] presented a similar application. But as these applications are designed for a small group of people, it is hard to deal with fast growing data.

In fact, most of dietary nutrition analysis methods face two issues need to solve. One issue is samples are not accurate, as most methods tend to use a sample got at a moment time to represent all samples produced during a period of time, which ignores

© Springer International Publishing AG 2016
X. Yin et al. (Eds.): HIS 2016, LNCS 10038, pp. 129–135, 2016.
DOI: 10.1007/978-3-319-48335-1_14

the fact samples may change over time. The other issue is the traditional data analysis methods is limited to process samples, as the number of samples is rapidly increasing and the types of samples are constantly emerging. Fortunately, the development of big data processing technologies provides a feasible base to solve the above issues. In this paper, a dietary nutrition analysis method is presented. This method takes advantage of *big data processing* to preprocess the samples to improve the quality of data, moreover, makes use of a parallelized *fuzzy clustering method leveraging Mapreduce* to complete the data analysis efficiently and effectively.

2 Motivation

In the Smart Campus System for Shaanxi Normal University (SNNU), there is a function that performs the dietary nutrition analysis for students, which can provide scientific guidance to keep the students healthy. If we use the traditional statistical analysis methods, some limitations need to add on samples. For example, for a kind of dishes, the nutrition keeps the same; even it is made of several ingredients. Obviously, this limitation is not reasonable. In fact, for the same dishes, each has different nutrition (the types of nutrition are the same but the values are various). Doing biochemical analysis for each dish every day needs lots of money and time, so it is impossible. How to solve this issue?

3 Preprocess by Big Data Processing

To improve the quality of data, this paper tries to make use of big data processing to obtain the data approximating the facts.

We utilize the following data:

(1) For each dish, the main ingredients and their quantity are known;
(2) For each ingredient, the nutrient contents are known;
(3) Usually, for each dish, the types of ingredient will not change, but the quantity may change to keep the same cost.

To keep the same cost, if the price of an ingredient increases, the quantity of the ingredient must decrease, vice versa. Obviously, the nutrition of each dish will fluctuate with price changes of the main ingredients.

We do the following works to preprocessing the data. Firstly, using a web crawler, the prices of ingredients can be obtained from Internet every day. Figure 1 shows the workflow of the crawler system. Then, by analyzing the obtained data weekly, we can get a variety of ingredients price which changes over time. For example, Fig. 2 gives the price curves of tomatoes and eggs in 2015. In addition, we could get the nutrient contents of some ingredients as Table 1 shows. According to Table 1, the standard nutrient of the dish can be obtained. Taking a dish of *tomato scrambled eggs* as an example, 200 g tomato and 100 g egg are needed. The standard nutrient of the dish is shown in Table 2.

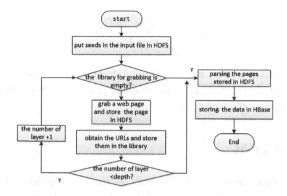

Fig. 1. The workflow of a crawler system

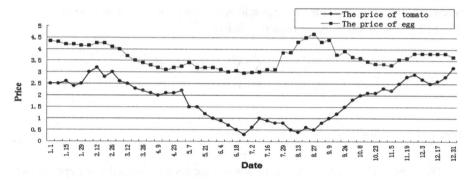

Fig. 2. The price curve of tomatoes and eggs in 2015

Table 1. The nutrients of 3 ingredients.

Nutrients	Tomato	Egg	Chicken
Pr. (g)	0.45	6.4	9.65
CAL (kcal)	9.50	78	83.5
Fat (g)	0.10	5.55	4.70
CHO (g)	2.00	0.65	0.65
Fiber (g)	0.25	-	-
VC (mg)	0.95	-	-
VE (mg)	0.29	1.15	0.36
Ca. (mg)	5.00	22.0	4.50

Table 2. The nutrients of 200 g tomato +100 g egg

Nutrients	Standard	2015/04/29	2015/09/03
Pr. (g)	14.60	15.88	15.13
CAL (kcal)	194.00	206.95	221.71
Fat (g)	11.50	12.81	10.42
CHO (g)	9.30	8.13	19.72
Fiber (g)	1.00	0.83	2.33
VC (mg)	3.80	3.17	8.84
VE (mg)	3.46	3.55	4.66
Ca. (mg)	64.00	66.10	84.12

Finally, according to the data model in Fig. 2, we can achieve that the price of tomatoes rose by 120 % and the price of egg dropped to 89 % on 2015/04/29, while the price of tomatoes dropped to 43 % and the price of egg rose by 117 % on 2015/09/03. The nutrients of the dish on 2015/04/29 and 2015/09/03, as shown in Table 2, are calculated by the following equations.

$$\text{nutrient} = \sum_{i=1}^{k} \frac{\alpha T_{wi}}{T_i(d)/T_{ai}} \tag{1}$$

Where, α is a nutrient containing in unit ingredient, T_{wi} is the quantity of the i ingredient containing in the dish, T_{ai} is the average price of the ingredient, and $T_t(d)$ is a function that maps a date to a price.

4 Parallelized FCM

The FCM algorithm attempts to partition a finite collection of n elements $X = \{x_1, \cdots, x_n\}$ into a collection of c fuzzy clusters with respect to some given criterion. Given a finite set of data, the algorithm returns a list of c cluster centers $C = \{c_1, \cdots, c_c\}$ and a partition matrix $W = \mu_{ij} \in [0, 1], i = 1, \cdots, n, j = 1, \cdots, c$, where each element, μ_{ij}, tells the degree to which element, x_i, belongs to cluster c_j. The FCM aims to minimize an objective function:

$$J(W, C) = \sum_{i=1}^{n} \sum_{j=1}^{c} \mu_{ij}^{m} ||x_i - c_j||^2 \tag{2}$$

Where $\mu_{ij} = \dfrac{1}{\sum_{k=1}^{c} (\frac{||x_i - c_j||}{||x_i - c_k||})^{2/(m-1)}}$ and $c_j = \dfrac{\sum_{j=1}^{n} (\mu_{ij})^m x_j}{\sum_{j=1}^{n} \mu_{ij}^m}$

The steps of FCM are as follows: (1) the parameters are assigned to the appropriate initial value, e.g., usually $m = 2$; (2) the cluster centers are initialized randomly; (3) the membership matrix W and the cluster centers C are updated, according to μ_{ij} and c_j; (4) according to the formula (2), the value of the objective function can be obtained; if the value is less than the threshold, the algorithm ends, else go to the step (3).

4.1 Parallelizing FCM by Mapreduce

This parallelized algorithm contains four main parts, i.e., Mapper, Combiner, Reducer, and Iteration.

Mapper

```
Input:  <key: line number, value: data >
Output: <key: cluster center ID, value: <data, degree of membership > >
```

The distance d_{ij} between a data $x_i(i = 1, \cdots, n)$ and a cluster center $c_j(j = 1, \cdots, c)$ is calculated so that the degree of membership μ_{ij} can be obtained. As a result, we obtain a partition matrix $W = \mu_{ij} \in [0, 1], i = 1, \cdots, n, j = 1, \cdots, c$.

Combiner

Input: < key: cluster center ID, value: <data, degree of membership >>
Output: < key: cluster center ID, value: <mapsum0, mapsum1 > >

In the Mapper module, the data size is $n \times c$. If the data size is huge, the bandwidth of network would become a bottleneck of data transmission. To solve this issue, two types of data are calculated as the following.

$$mapsum0[i] = \sum_{j=1}^{n} \mu_{ij}^{m}, (i = 1, \cdots, c) \tag{3}$$

$$mapsum1[i] = \sum_{j=1}^{n} \mu_{ij}^{m} x_j, (i = 1, \cdots, c) \tag{4}$$

Reducer

Input: < key: cluster center ID, value: <mapsum0, mapsum1 >>
Output: < key: cluster center ID, value: <cluster center > >

In the Reducer module, the cluster center is updated as the following and the new cluster centers are stored in a file named *newCenterFile*.

$$c_i = \sum_{i=1}^{c} mapsum1[i] / \sum_{i=1}^{c} mapsum0[i], (i = 1, \cdots, c) \tag{5}$$

Iteration

This Iteration module is used to determine whether the cluster center convergence. This module compares the number of iteration and the threshold. If the number of iteration is greater than the threshold, this parallelized FCM end, else this module compares two files (one is the *newCenterFile* and the other is *oldCenterFile*), if the they are same, or there are $(c_i' = c_i)$ *or* $(|c_i' - c_i| < threshold)$, where $i = 1, \cdots, c$, $c_i' \in C_{old}, c_i \in C_{new}$, this parallelized FCM end, else *oldCenterFile* is overwritten by *newCenterFile* and iterative process continues.

4.2   Selecting Clustering Centers

If we use the annual average prices of ingredients as the baseline to estimate the change of ingredient prices, it leads to larger changes of nutrition for dishes, which makes the data to be analyzed more dispersed. As a result, the data analysis may be affected due to some sensitive data.

Therefore, we do the following works to solve this problem. First, the data are divided into four parts (as the price changes are smeller in the same season), and the average price of an ingredient in a season is adopted as the baseline to estimate the price changes of the ingredient. Second, by analyzing the prices, we can identify some ingredients largely supplied in the season. Finally, we find all of dishes related with the ingredients and calculate the average nutrients of the dishes. The values are used to select the cluster centers. We set 3 clusters. One cluster center adopts the data that is the same as the average nutrients, one employs the data lower than the average nutrients, and another utilizes the data higher than the average nutrients.

5 Experiment

This experiment takes the dining data of 28,000 students in Shaanxi Normal University in 2015 as samples. We know what dishes a student ate and how much to eat. The procedure of the experiment is as follows: (1) data preprocessing is done; (2) selecting cluster centers; (3) analyzing data by the parallelized FCM.

This experiment takes the Chinese Dietary Reference Intakes [1] as the baseline to estimate whether the students have rational dietary intakes. The advice of dietary nutrients intakes for a student in the spring is shown in Table 3. We can obtain the average dairy nutrients intakes for a studentby the following equation, where w_i equals the ratio of the number of students belonging to a cluster center and the total number of students.

$$average\ nutrients\ intakes = \sum_{i=1}^{c} w_i c_i \qquad (6)$$

Table 3. The dietary nutrients intakes for a student (Jan to Mar, 2015)

Nutrients	Baseline	Center 1	Center 2	Center 3	Average	Status
Pr. (g)	70	75.25	69.25	80.24	74.98	↑
CAL (kcal)	2250	2158.35	1860.45	2891.47	2060.72	↓
Fat (g)	62.5	60.59	51.32	87.38	59.05	↓
CHO (g)	337.5	296.37	250.48	384.12	279.65	↓
Fiber (g)	28	12.3	10.56	16.87	11.82	↓
VC (mg)	100	185.84	172.3	155.86	159.34	↑
VE (mg)	14	15.83	13.24	14.48	13.65	≈
Ca. (mg)	800	375.26	388.79	425.37	349.88	↓

6 Conclusion

In this paper, a dietary nutrition analysis mehtod is presented. On the one hand, the data are preprocessed leveraging big data processing, to approximate the facts. On the other hand, the data analysis method are improved in the performance by Mapreduce, to solve the issue that the number of samples is rapidly increasing. Finally, the experiments prove that this method is practible.

Acknowledgments. This paper is supported by the National Natural Science Foundation of China (NO. 11271237) and by the Fundamental Research Funds for the Central Universities (GK201603086).

References

1. Jiang, J., et al.: Dietary intake of human essential elements from a total diet study in Shenzhen, Guangdong Province. China. J. Food Compos. Anal. **39**, 1–7 (2015)
2. Magge, H., Sprinz, P., Adams, W.G., Drainoni, M.L., Meyers, A.: Zinc protoporphyrin and iron deficiency screening: trends and therapeutic response in an urban pediatric center. JAMA Pediatr. **167**(4), 361–367 (2013)
3. Zhu, S.: Dietary surveys by microcomputer. J. Harbin Med. Univ. (3), 56–58 (1987)
4. Zhang, J., Liao, H.: Micro-computer applications for dietary assessment. J. Fujian Med. Coll. **20**(1), 62–65 (1987)

Autism Spectrum Disorder:
Brain Images and Registration

Porawat Visutsak[1,2(✉)] and Yan Li[2]

[1] Department of Computer and Information Science, Faculty of Applied Science,
King Mongkut's University of Technology North Bangkok (KMUTNB),
Bangkok, Thailand
[2] Faculty of Health, Engineering and Sciences,
University of Southern Queensland, Toowoomba, Queensland, Australia
{porawat.visutsak,yan.li}@usq.edu.au

Abstract. Autism is a disorder of brain function that results in languages, communications, social interactions, behaviors, and interests. Various studies of autism in the field of neuroscience and computer science have introduced the complexity of this developmental disability by analyzing nerve signal and brain images. This paper presents the study of the abnormalities in autistic brain images using a new image registration method called "Template-based affine registration". The major contribution of this technique is aligning the different set of brain images, captured from different devices into a new coordinate system. By using the homogeneous coordinate transformation, the new method provides a robust transformation against rotation and translations of source and target images. The implementation of this study in autistic brain images yields the good results.

Keywords: Autism · Medical imaging · Brain images · Registration · Image processing

1 Introduction

In this section, the term of autism spectrum disorder and a general overview of the developmental disability are provided. Autism can be defined as a group of children who have severe social, language, and communication problems. This developmental disability leads to social isolation which is the name of 'autism' originated ('aut' means self, therefore 'autism' being removed from social interaction and communication). Autism may also be referred to conditions where somebody might be removed from social interaction and communication, leaving them alone or isolated [1].

American Psychiatric Association (APA) has been given the standard classification of mental disorders used by mental health professionals in the United States, called the diagnostic and statistical manual for mental disorders (DSM). DSM is intended to be used in all clinical settings by clinicians of different theoretical orientations. This standard can be used by mental health and other health professionals, including psychiatrists and other physicians, psychologists, social workers, nurses, occupational and rehabilitation therapists, and counselors.

© Springer International Publishing AG 2016
X. Yin et al. (Eds.): HIS 2016, LNCS 10038, pp. 136–146, 2016.
DOI: 10.1007/978-3-319-48335-1_15

In 2013, the DSM-V, a new revised DSM edition has been given the severity scores in each area which can help determine how much support the children are going to need [2–7], e.g. severity Level 1 indicates the children need some support, such as for social communication. They might be given full sentences for engaging a communication because normal conversations don't seem to work for repetitive and restrictive behaviors. They might have difficulties in switching activities (Fig. 1 shows the severity level of ASD). On the other side of spectra, on Level 3 severity, it indicates the children need a substantial support. In the social communication side, they might have only few words to speak and rarely initiate an interaction with others. For repetitive and restrictive behaviors, they might be extremely resistant to change and interferes seriously with daily life (Table 1 shows the details of each severity level).

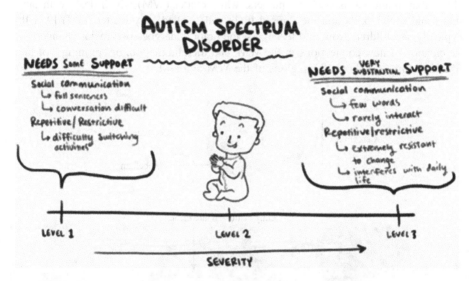

Fig. 1. The severity level of ASD (http://open.osmosis.org, retrieved 12 May 2016)

There are more accurate and medically useful ways for the diagnosis of individuals. For example, those previously described as Asperger's syndrome would likely fall closely to severity Level 1 than to severity Level 3. Much research to study the causes of autism have been reported, but the understanding of the theory of causation of autism and the other ASD is still incomplete [8]. Generally speaking, ASD starts with a genetic cause which ultimately affects the brain's development, specifically those relevant to the areas of social and communication behaviors. Which gene or the combination of genes that effects on ASD is still very much mysterious. Initially, there are a bunch of environmental triggers that have to be explored, but so far, there have been no clear risk factors that have been identified. There are no cures for ASD, and treatment or management have to be specifically and carefully tailored to each child. These include special educational programs and behavior therapies that seem to maximize the quality of life and functional independency.

Table 1. The details of each severity level

Severity	Social communication and interaction deficits	Restricted or repetitive behaviour
1	Full sentences Conversation difficulties	Difficulties with switching activities
2	In Between - Not specified (depends on each type of PDDs)	
3	Few words Rarely interacting	Extremely resistant to change Interferes with daily life

2 Autistic Brain Images

The human brain consists of two matters: white matter (WM) which deals with language and social skills and the unused brain cells, called gray matter (GM) [9, 10]. Typically, as children grow into teenagers, the brain undergoes two major changes — the creation of new connections in the WM, and the elimination, or "pruning," of the GM [11]. Figure 2 shows the regions of the WM and GM.

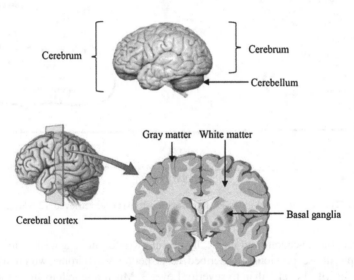

Fig. 2. The connections between the WM and GM and Cerebral cortex (http://www.bioon.com/book/biology/whole/image/1/1-6.tif.jpg, retrieved 13 May 2016)

In Fig. 2, the major brain regions implicated in autism have been investigated [12]: 1. Cerebral cortex (social impairment, communication deficits and repetitive behaviors): a thin layer of gray matter on the surface of the cerebral hemispheres. Two-thirds of its area are deep in the fissures (deep grooves, generally dividing large regions/lobes of the brain) or folds. Cerebrum is responsible for mental functions, general movement, perception, and behavioral reactions. If the area in the frontal lobe of cerebrum is damaged, one may have difficulty in speaking and writing, e.g. the individual may speak in long sentences that have no meaning, add unnecessary words, and even create new words. 2. Cerebellum, located at the back of the brain, it fine tunes brain activities, regulates balances, body movements, coordination and the muscles used in speaking. 3. Basal ganglia (communication deficits and repetitive behaviors, Basal ganglia helps regulate automatic movement): gray masses deep in the cerebral hemisphere that serves as a connection between the cerebrum and cerebellum. 4. Corpus callosum: consists primarily of closely packed bundles of fibers that connect the right and left hemispheres and allows for communications between the hemispheres. 5. Brain stem, located in the front of the cerebellum: it serves as a relay station, passing messages between various parts of the body and the cerebral cortex. Primary functions are the heart rate control and breathing. Figure 3 shows corpus callosum and brain stem.

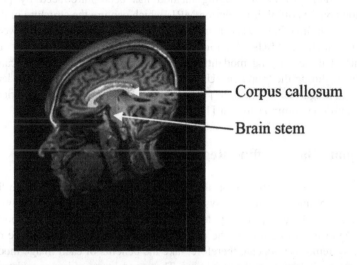

Fig. 3. Vertical MRI scanning (Corpus callosum and Brain stem) [14]

To study the brain activities related to brain regions previously described, various image modalities have been applied such as T1-weighted MRI (Magnetic Resonance Imaging), the Brain-Wide Association Analysis (BWAS), and the multi-modality of brain imaging method. The latest T1-MRI modality proposed by [10] is used to monitor the structure of autistic brain images during treatments. To study how the brain of autism changes over time, researchers captured the brain images of children with autism before the treatment (in some cases, before attending special educational courses for autistic children) and they captured similar images again approximately three years later. By repeating imaging with the benefit of T1-MRI, the scientists would see the before and after images of brain regions which correspond to autisms' deficits, therefore they can create a detailed picture of how their brains change over times. Thus, this new knowledge may help explain some of the symptoms of autism and could improve future treatment options later on [11]. The major drawback of T1-MRI modality is the lack of useful information for the brain activity analysis, which is required for individual diagnosis in order to understand the deficits (social impairment, communication deficits and repetitive behaviors), which are the problems of children with ASD.

The modified version of fMRI (Functional Magnetic Resonance Imaging) modality has been proposed by [13]. The BWAS is the big data concept-based computation. The major task of the BWAS is used to analyze fMRI of autistic brain scans with the capacity of creating the panoramic views of the whole brain from the real time manipulating of one billion pieces of data. The system also provides a 3D model of autistic brain which is very useful for scientists. The ability to analyze the entire data set from a bunch of fMRI scans provided the authors the opportunity to compile, compare and contrast accurate imaging modalities for both autistic (a study group) and non-autistic brains (a control group) [11]. The cost of computation and resources of the hardware to handle the big data are the factors which should be taking into account. The multi-modality of brain imaging method has been introduced by [14]. This combination consists of: high-resolution MRIs which capture the structure of the brain; Diffusion Tensor Imaging (DTI), a method to trace the connections between brain regions; and functional MRIs which indicate brain activity [11]. Researchers can gain the benefits of three imaging modalities by observing the autistic brain scans at the different times during the treatment. Unfortunately, they have to do these at least three times per one diagnosis. Visutsak in [14] explained how to combine the various types of images into one common format [11].

3   Template-Based Affine Registration

Image registration is the process of aligning the different sets of data from the same object into a common coordinate system, aligning them in order to analyze subtle changes among each other [15]. A potential application, which plays an important role in ASD diagnosis, is to combine the different brain image modals into one common coordinate system. Doctors can, therefore, take the benefits of each image modality by observing the brain images at the same time. The general term of image registration can be defined as the evolution of a source image to a target image. This evolution refers to as a proper mapping function being used to spatially transform two images with respect to their intensities [15]. Once the mapping function is determined, the alignment step can be accomplished using the warping. Thus the source and target images are aligned properly. The following equations show the definition of image registration derived from [11, 15]:

Assume the mapping function is a polynomial of order N, by identifying $K \geq N$ corresponding points between the source and target images, we have:

$$(u_i, v_i) \leftrightarrow (x_i, \ y_i), \ i = 1, \ 2 \ldots, K \tag{1}$$

Determine the coefficients a_i, b_i, $i = 0, \ldots, N-1$ by solving,

$$\begin{aligned} x(u_i, v_i) &= a_0 + a_1 u_i + a_2 v_i + \ldots = x_i \\ y(u_i, v_i) &= b_0 + b_1 u_i + b_2 v_i + \ldots = y_i \end{aligned} \tag{2}$$

$i = 1, \ 2 \ldots, K$. Suppose, Aa = x, Ab = y,
where

$$A = \begin{bmatrix} 1 & u_1 & v_1 & \cdots \\ 1 & u_2 & v_2 & \cdots \\ \vdots & \vdots & \vdots & \ddots \\ 1 & u_k & v_k & \cdots \end{bmatrix}, a = \begin{bmatrix} a_0 \\ a_1 \\ \vdots \\ a_{N-1} \end{bmatrix}, b = \begin{bmatrix} b_0 \\ b_1 \\ \vdots \\ b_{N-1} \end{bmatrix}, x = \begin{bmatrix} x_1 \\ x_2 \\ \vdots \\ x_k \end{bmatrix}, y = \begin{bmatrix} y_1 \\ y_2 \\ \vdots \\ y_k \end{bmatrix} \quad (3)$$

A is the affine transformation matrix. The term "Template" means the point set extracted from the source image. The goal is to estimate the affine transformation for the source and target images using two point sets extracted from these two images [11]. In order to use an affine mapping to register images, three or more pairs of corresponding points are needed. To solve Eq. (3), it is straightforward by using three pairs of points. Usually, it is recommended to use more than three pairs to obtain the best fitting affine parameters (these pairs may not all be related by an affine mapping, finding the linear least square fit by solving an over-determined system of equations is more practical).

Given two brain images, to register one with the other can be done by manually marking corresponding points, ideally, chosen by doctors among the interested points such as the features in the major brain regions implicated in ASD (see Sect. 2 for details). Figure 4 shows the registration of brain images.

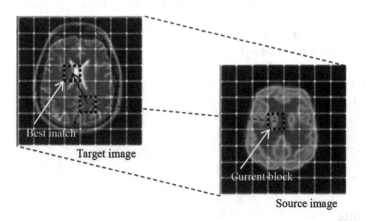

Fig. 4. Image registration (put a small block around the point in the source image, then find a block in target image that matches the block pattern the best. The process involves exhaustive search within a certain range)

By given a threshold value (T), the algorithm is applied to find the transformation having the best linear least square fit, the three parameters of affine transformation are θ, t_x, and t_y (rotation and translation in x-y axis) which are denoted by d_θ, d_{tx}, and d_{ty}, respectively. The transformation algorithm is as follows:

```
Assign the initial values: θ₁ ∈ Tθ, tₓ₁ ∈ Tₓ, ty₂ ∈ Ty;
Where Tθ = {θ - dθ, θ, θ + dθ}
      Tₓ = {tₓ - dtₓ, tₓ, tₓ + dtₓ}
      Ty = {ty - dty, ty, ty + dty}
Set the number of the iterations: iteration = 5;
for i = 1 to iteration;
  temp_θ = [θ; θ - dθ; θ + dθ];
    for loop_θ = 1 to size(temp_θ);
      temp_tₓ = [tₓ; tₓ - dtₓ; tₓ + dtₓ];
        for loop_tₓ = 1 to size(temp_tₓ);
          temp_ty = [ty; ty - dty; ty + dty];
            for loop_ty = 1 to size(temp_ty);
              -Two images are transformed by (temp_θ(
              loop_θ), temp_tₓ(loop_tₓ), temp_ty(loop_ty))
              -Compute the linear least square fit: LS
              if LS is lower than Previous_LS then
                set the best transformation to the current
                transformation:
                  best_θ = temp_θ(loop_θ);
                  best_tₓ= temp_tₓ(loop_tₓ);
                  best_ty= temp_ty(loop_ty);
              end for loop_ty
          end for loop_tₓ
      end for loop_θ
  Update the values:
    θ = best_θ;
    tₓ = best_tₓ;
    ty = best_ty;
end for
```

4 Results

The major contribution of this study has been modified from [11]. Instead of using 6–12 landmark points in source and target images (the conventional method), this study used the control block together with the linear least square fit computation to find the affine mapping function. The study used the autistic brain image datasets from [16]. The selected images in both MRIs and DTIs were used as the source and target images, respectively. The study involves integrating the images to create a composite view. Extracting the useful information is helpful for further studying ASD. The study yielded good results with a reasonable cost of computation. Figure 6 shows the results of image registration (conventional brain magnetic resonance images (MRIs) and diffusion tensor images (DTIs) of a patient (13-month-old male)).

The registration results are evaluated in qualitative and quantitative evaluations. The qualitative evaluation is performed by visually compare the location of edge in grid (see Figs. 4 and 5), whereas the quantitative evaluation is performed as follows:

- Manually draw the edge of the object in both source and target images.
- For each edge pixel in the source image, calculate the distance to the nearest edge pixel in the target image.
- Calculate the mean and the maximum distance with the following equations:

$$\text{Maximum dist.} = Max(d_i) \tag{4}$$

where d_i = the distance between the edge pixel i in the source image and the nearest edge pixel in the target image (see Fig. 4)

$$\text{Mean dist.} = \frac{\sum_{i=1}^{N} d_i}{n} \tag{5}$$

where n = the number of edge pixels

Table 2 shows the maximum and the mean distances of the test image (the conventional method and the proposed method). The proposed method gave the both values (the maximum and the mean distances) lower than the conventional method. The major concern for the visual perception (the qualitative evaluation) is that even though the distances indicate the correctness of the registration, the lower value does not imply the better quality of image visualization in human eyes. Figure 5 shows the registered outline and the overlapped images of the proposed method.

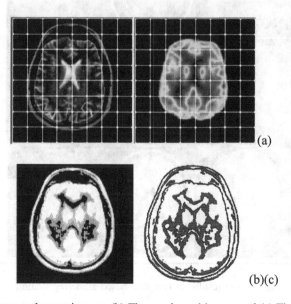

Fig. 5. (a) Source and target images, (b) The overlapped image, and (c) The outline image

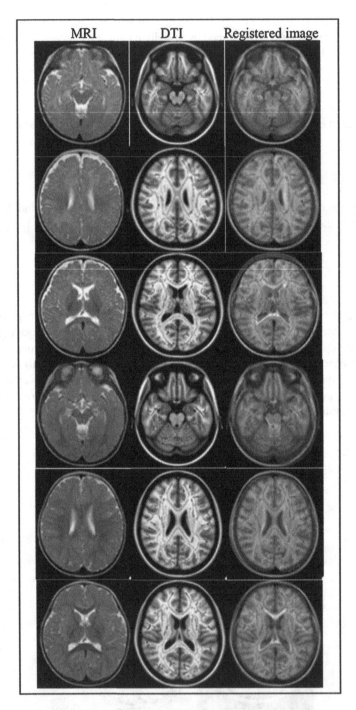

Fig. 6. The results of Template-based affine registration

Table 2. The maximum and the mean distances of the test image (the conventional method and the proposed method)

Test image		Conventional registration method	Proposed registration method
Image skull (Fig. 5)	Maximum dist.	39.43	21.08
	Mean dist.	8.34	2.92

*Note that: the maximum and the mean distances of the result images in Fig. 6 are omitted since the test objects in this paper are skull and brain images, therefore the maximum and mean distances are not varied.

5   Conclusions

This study presents an important matter in image registration. The study is helpful to register two multimodalities of autistic brain images. The experiments demonstrate that the method yields a good affine mapping function and it also gives the good resolution images as well as the optimal running times. The limitation of this work is the lack of datasets since the study needs the test images in both formats of MRIs and DTIs for registration.

Acknowledgements. "This research was funded by the King Mongkut's University of Technology North Bangkok. Contract no. KMUTNB-GOV-59-30". We would also like to thank the Endeavour Research Fellowship Programme and the Australian Government for financial support during the study at the University of Southern Queensland.

References

1. Rapin, I., Tuchman, R.F.: Autism: definition, neurobiology, screening, diagnosis. Pediatr. Clin. North Am. **55**(5), 1129–1146 (2008). doi:10.1016/j.pcl.2008.07.005
2. Johnson, C.P., Myers, S.M.: Identification and evaluation of children with autism spectrum disorders. Pediatrics **120**(5), 1183–1215 (2007). doi:10.1542/peds.2007-2361
3. American Psychiatric Association: Diagnostic and statistical manual of mental disorders: DSM-IV, 4th edn. American Psychiatric Association, Washington, DC (2000). ISBN 978-0-89042-025-6
4. McPartland, J., Volkmar, F.R.: Autism and related disorders. Handb. Clin. Neurol. **106**, 407–418 (2012). doi:10.1016/B978-0-444-52002-9.00023-1
5. Venkat, A., Jauch, E., Russell, W.S., Crist, C.R., Farrell, R.: Care of the patient with an autism spectrum disorder by the general physician. Postgrad. Med. J. **88**(1042), 472–481 (2012). doi:10.1136/postgradmedj-2011-130727
6. American Psychiatric Association: Diagnostic and statistical manual of mental disorders: DSM-V. 5th edn. American Psychiatric Association, Washington, DC (2013). ISBN 978-0-89042-554-1
7. Handbook of Autism and Pervasive Developmental Disorders, Assessment, Interventions, and Policy. John Wiley & Sons (2014). ISBN 1-118-28220-5 (2016). Retrieved 12 May 2016

8. Trottier, G., Srivastava, L., Walker, C.D.: Etiology of infantile autism: a review of recent advances in genetic and neurobiological research. J. Psychiatry Neurosci. **24**(2), 103–115 (1999)

9. Fahmi, R., et al.: Structural MRI-based discrimination between autistic and typically developing brain. In: Proceedings of Computer Assisted Radiology and Surgery (CARS 2007), Berlin, Germany, pp. 24–26 (2007)

10. Christopher, F.: Autistic Brains Develop More Slowly Than Healthy Brains. BMED Report, 28 October 2011

11. Porawat, V.: Template-based affine registration of autistic brain images. In: Proceedings of the 7th International Joint Conference on Computational Intelligence, IJCCI 2015, Lisbon Marriott Hotel, Lisbon, Portugal, 12–14 November, vol. 2, pp. 188–192 (2015)

12. Amaral, D.G., Schumann, C.M., Nordahl, C.W.: Neuroanatomy of autism. Trends Neurosci. **31**(3), 137–145 (2008). doi:10.1016/j.tins.2007.12.005

13. Cheng, W., et al.: Autism: reduced connectivity between cortical areas involved with face expression, theory of mind, and the sense of self. Brain, A Journal of Neurology (2015). Oxford University Press

14. Virginia, H.: Researchers reveals first brain study of Temple Grandin. The 2012 Society for Neuroscience annual meeting, Simons Foundation Autism Research Initiative (SFARI), 14 October 2012

15. Porawat, V.: Multi-grid transformation for medical image registration. In: 2014 International Conference on Advanced Computer Science and Information Systems, Ambhara Hotel, Blok M, Jakarta, Indonesia, 18–19 October, pp. 52–56 (2014)

16. http://fcon_1000.projects.nitrc.org/indi/abide/. Retrieved 11 Jan 2015

Study on Intelligent Home Care Platform Based on Chronic Disease Knowledge Management

Ye Chen[1] and Hao Fan[2(✉)]

[1] Center for the Studies of Information Resources, Wuhan University,
Wuhan 430072, P.R. China
[2] School of Information Management, Wuhan University, Wuhan 430072, P.R. China
hfan@whu.edu.cn

Abstract. As the elderly population has been rapidly expanding, needs of adequate health and housing services for elderly people continue to grow, but resources for providing such services are becoming increasingly scarce. Thus, using modern technologies and efficiently providing Intelligent Home Care (IHC) services is regarded as a pressing issue. In order to handle issues of the coming aging society, this article analyzes health monitoring, health prevention, health advisor and knowledge service requirements of an IHC Platform, and proposes an architecture of the IHC Platform based on chronic disease knowledge management, which is excepted to offer intelligent, accurate and personal care service for elderly people.

Keywords: Intelligent Home Care · Chronic disease · Knowledge management · Platform framework

1 Introduction

With the elderly population steadily growing, issues of health care are widely concerned by society researchers. The report, *Development of Chinese Aging*, states that the number of population aged over 60 has reached 202 million in China, the population aging level has reached 14.8 % by the end of 2013 [1]. Meanwhile, morbidity rates of chronic diseases, such as coronary heart diseases, hypertension, diabetes, asthma and arthritis, among people over 65 is 3 − 7 times more than younger ones aged from 15 to 45 [2]. The arrival of an aging society brings serious challenges to health care services. More medical facilities are required, such as hospitals and health recovery centers, to meet health care needs of the elderly. Also, it is difficult for families with common incomes to gain health care services due to the limited and costly medical resources. Furthermore, elderly people might prefer to receive health care services living at home.

This paper is supported by the Chinese NSFC International Cooperation and Exchange Program, *Research on Intelligent Home Care Platform based on Chronic Diseases Knowledge Management* (71661167007).

X. Yin et al. (Eds.): HIS 2016, LNCS 10038, pp. 147–153, 2016.
DOI: 10.1007/978-3-319-48335-1_16

In this sense, Intelligent Home Care (IHC) services can be a solution to the described problems. With the development of technologies acquiring medical and health information by portable devices, a large number of medical and individual health data is generated, which makes the health status monitoring possible. In the meantime, medical research literatures, health care knowledge, and clinical case data about chronic diseases are widely distributed on Internet, specialist clinic data sets, books and other places. All the information could be the data sources of a chronic disease knowledge base. Therefore, rapid developments of mobile Internet, wearable devices and big data technologies bring the chance to set up an IHC system based on chronic disease knowledge management, so that people can get health care services either at home or in communities. Our research is to analyze the requirements of an IHC for elderly people and design a IHC platform based on chronic disease knowledge management.

The remainder of this paper is organized as follows. In Sect. 2, we present related work. Section 3 analyzes requirements of an IHC Platform, and Sect. 4 describes the framework of the IHC platform based on chronic disease knowledge management. Section 5 contains conclusions and future work.

2   Related Work

Intelligent Home Care is a new concept aiming to help elderly people and improve their life quality either at home or in communities, which makes them not to be constrained by time and geographical environments in daily life. Based on the foundation of the Internet of things, intelligent cloud computing and other technologies, IHC is to achieve a seamless connection among all kinds of sensor terminals and computer networks [3].

In recent research, the problem of combining artificial intelligence and operational technologies, such as sensors, actuators, communications, and ubiquitous computing, for assisting people's daily life within a spread environment has become an emerging research topic, as known as *Ambient Intelligence*(AmI)[4]. A typical context of applying ambient intelligence technologies is in smart home environments [5]. Techniques, such as wireless technologies, mobile tools, wearable instruments, intelligent artifacts, handhold devices, etc., can professionally improve the efficiency of health care task manage and increase the quality of patient care [6]. Su and Chiang [7] propose an *Ambient Intelligent Community Care Platform* (AICCP) by applying Radio-Frequency Identification (RFID) and Mobile Agent technologies to enable the care givers and communities to offer pervasive and context-aware care services. Zhu [8] designs a smart pension service platform based on wearable device, which uses multiple sensor nodes to collect data and transmit it into the central node through the ZigBee network, then uses GSM/GPRS wireless communication modules transmitting the data to the service center, in order to achieve the objective of real-time services.

The imbalances and differences of medical diagnosis and treatment among regions and medical institutions make it unable for many patients to access a high level of standard health care, and it is also difficult to effectively guarantee medical qualities. In order to meet various demands of intelligent health care systems, technologies of knowledge-based systems have advantages in extensibility and flexibility, which can be widely used in practical applications, including clinical decision supporting and health care information systems [10].

Ontology-based computational models have been proposed to facilitate effective management and acquisition of medical knowledge [9], and to be treated as a foundation of medical diagnosis and treatment [11]. Su and Peng address ontological and epistemological issues of information services through the example of OntoRis, which is an ontology-based rehabilitation service designed to assist patients in acquiring practicable knowledge about the prescribed rehabilitation activities, and expedite their recovery by providing suggestions and advices drawn from the evidence-based medicine [12]. Chen et al. [13] provide an framework of intelligent knowledge-based and customizable home care system with ubiquitous patient monitoring and alerting techniques.

In order to fulfill extensible, personalized and intelligent demands of elderly people, who may have different health and disease conditions in various living environments, this study investigates an approach integrating chronic disease knowledge bases and personal health databases to construct an IHC platform based on the combination of Ambient Intelligence and knowledge-based system technologies.

3   Requirements of Intelligent Home Care Platform

IHC platform users may include individual persons and patients, health care experts, medical institutions, etc. Due to the diversification and individuation of user demands, the platform is concerned with multiple function models, including health monitoring, health prevention, health advisor and knowledge service.

(1) **Health Monitoring.** Health monitoring is a process of collecting and storing health data, and used to reflect person's health condition from different aspects, such as physical examination results, daily monitoring data and clinical medical records. The real-time monitoring and feedback of person's health status aims to achieve all-time emergency services, which is also the basis of timely prevention and accurate health advices.

(2) **Health Prevention.** Health prevention is one of the vital requirements of the IHC platform for the elderly. Prevention is much more important than treatment, which aims to stop disease before it starts, or to detect risk factors. It could be also used to prevent diseases by detecting implicit symptoms for asymptomatic people, and help them to be treated early. In addition, the pathogeny of chronic diseases is usually formed by long-term accumulation of unhealthy lifestyles. It is not easy to aware changes of a body before the onset of a disease. Health condition prevention and family pathological analysis play a significant role in keeping healthy and living a better life.

(3) **Health Advisor.** Health advisor is to provide services of maintaining elderly people's physical condition and lifestyle at a healthy level and helping them to alleviate discomforts and symptoms of diseases. Providing health advices is a fundamental requirement of the IHC platform, which may contain two aspects: health care advices and treatment advices, such as health guideline, comprehensive treatments, and accurate medical procedures.

(4) **Knowledge Service.** In daily life, elderly people might encounter various health problems such as indigestion, insomnia, body ache, cold fever and so on. They require reliable and trusted knowledge about health care and disease to help themselves for treatments. Furthermore, due to the influence of gene, similar life habit and other factors, people within a family seem to have the same diseases, pathological features and treatment response. Health education and counseling of a family, including chronic disease, daily life care, family health management, etc., are able to enhance the health self-management ability of the family.

4   Framework of Intelligent Home Care Platform

In order to satisfy the requirements mentioned in Sect. 3, we propose an Intelligent Home Care Platform to support the accomplishment of multi-form applications, which consists of four layers: Data Layer, System Layer, Service Layer and Application Layer, as shown in Fig. 1.

The **Data Layer** extracts chronic disease knowledge from distributed sources and collects various types of personal health data. The data source of the IHC platform includes medical research literatures, medical indicator systems, health

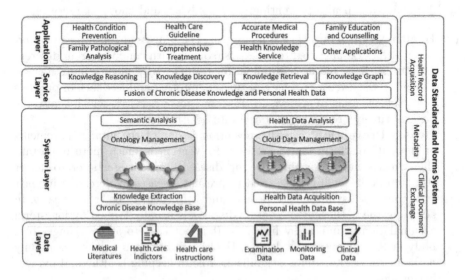

Fig. 1. The Intelligent Home Care Platform architecture

care knowledge instructions, and so on, to provide original information for constructing chronic disease knowledge bases in the upper System Layer. It also includes physical examination results, daily monitoring data and clinical medical records, which are data sources of personal health database.

The **System Layer** is the core portion of the platform, which consists of functional systems managing two bases, i.e. the chronic disease knowledge base and the personal health database. The knowledge base system extracts specific knowledge of particular chronic disease, e.g. hypertension, and uses ontology to organize and manage these knowledge in order to provide functional supports of semantic analysis and modelling for the knowledge services, such as knowledge reasoning and knowledge retrieval. The personal database is considered to be organized and managed by the way of cloud storage, in order to handle the problem of a large number of medical and personal health data generated by the modern technologies acquiring medical and health data of individuals.

The **Service Layer** is the connection between the System Layer and the Application Layer, including modules providing functionalities of knowledge retrieval, reasoning and discovering, which is based on the fusion of chronic disease knowledge and personal health data. When platform users need to access specific knowledge contents and instances of the knowledge base, user queries are decomposed, step by step, into various specific sub-queries over the chronic disease knowledge sources, and knowledge retrieval module acquires query results from the source in manners of stream or batch processing. Knowledge reasoning and discovering modules acquire latent semantic information of chronic disease and health knowledge concepts by using logical reasoning, which meets the demand of semantic revealing and computer interactive to the platform.

The **Application Layer** is the interface of the IHC Platform, which provides various kinds of health care services. Health condition prevention achieves all-day emergency and warning service based on monitoring user health situation and its feedback; Family pathological analysis aims to analyze family pathologic features, drug effects, and discomfort reactions for user diagnosis and treatment decision; Health care guideline leads users to live in a more health and scientific lifestyle and protect people against chronic diseases; Comprehensive treatments mean that taking care about patient needs as a whole, not just medical and physical sides, and providing health services as the same provided by many professionals working together; Accurate medical procedures are involved in the platform to maximize positive effects and minimize side ones of treatments to achieve personalized IHC; Health knowledge service mainly provides causes, symptoms, diagnosis of chronic diseases to users; Family health education and counseling is able to enhance health self-management abilities of families.

Key issues of constructing the IHC Platform lay on knowledge-based reasoning mechanism, and depend on chronic disease knowledge and health databases. The requirements of health monitoring, prevention and advisor can not be fulfilled only by crawling relative information from web pages or combining materials scattered in different databases together. Knowledge reasoning, discovery, retrieval and knowledge graph techniques are used for realizing the requirements.

Meanwhile, in order to efficiently invoke and sequentially communicate between adjacent layers, such as the Data Layer and the System Layer, data standard and norm systems are considered to standardize representation, transformation, and inter-operation procedures of medical data, such as health record acquisition, meta data management, clinical document exchange, etc.

5   Conclusion and Future Work

With the coming of aging society, issues of home care have aroused wide concern in research. Elderly people with different health and disease conditions have different requirements. This paper analyzes requirements for designing an IHC platform. Various requirements including health monitoring, health prevention, health advisor and knowledge service are considered, and a four-layer architecture, i.e. the Data, System, Service and Application Layer, of the IHC platform is concerned to satisfy the extensible, personalized and intelligent demands of home care. In constructing the platform, knowledge fusion is used for establishing semantic associations between chronic disease knowledge and personal health data. The future work will focus on developing knowledge fusion methods and implementing the platform in a specific chronic disease domain.

References

1. Chinese Academy of Social Sciences: The development of Chinese Aging [EB, OL], May 2016. http://www.360doc.com/content/14/0331/20/8290311_365284728. shtml
2. Li, G., Cong, Y.: Discussion of comprehensive prevention mode of chronic noncommunicable diseases. China Health Ind. **12**(17), 177–179 (2015)
3. Xi, H., Ren, X., Qu, S.: Smart pension: the elderly care service innovation with information technology. Sci. Res. Aging **2**(7), 12–21 (2015)
4. Ramos, C., Augusto, J., Shapiro, D.: Ambient intelligencethe next step for artificial intelligence. IEEE Intell. Syst. **23**(2), 15–18 (2008)
5. Bielikov, M., Krajcovic, T.: Ambient intelligence within a home environment. ERCIM News **47**, 12–13 (2001)
6. Bricon-Souf, N., Newman, C.: Context awareness in health care: a review. Int. J. Med. Informatics **76**(1), 2–12 (2007)
7. Su, C., Chiang, C.: Pervasive community care platform: ambient Intelligence leveraging sensor networks and mobile agents. Int. J. Syst. Sci. **45**(4), 778–797 (2014)
8. Zhu, J.: Construction of the service platform for smart pension based on wearable device. Softw. Eng. **19**(1), 39–41 (2016)
9. Juarez, J., Riestra, T., Campos, M., et al.: Medical knowledge management for specific hospital departments. Expert Syst. Appl. **36**(10), 12214–12224 (2009)
10. Wang, W., Cheung, C., Lee, W., Kwok, S.: Knowledge based treatment planning for adolescent early intervention of mental healthcare: a hybrid case based reasoning approach. Expert Syst. **24**(4), 232–251 (2007)
11. Garca-Crespo, À., Rodríguez, A., Mencke, M., et al.: ODDIN: Ontology-driven differential diagnosis based on logical inference and probabilistic refinements. Expert Syst. Appl. **37**(3), 2621–2628 (2010)

12. Su, C., Peng, C.: Multi-agent ontology-based Web 2.0 platform for medical reha-
    bilitation. Expert Syst. Appl. **39**(12), 10311–10323 (2012)
13. Chen, Y., Chiang, H., Yu, C., et al.: An intelligent knowledge-based and customiz-
    able home care system framework with ubiquitous patient monitoring and alerting
    techniques. Sensors **12**(8), 11154–11186 (2012)
14. Luijkx, K., Peek, S., Wouters, E.: Older adults and the role of family members in
    their acceptance of technology. Int. J. Environ. Res. public Health **12**(12), 15470–
    15485 (2015)

An Architecture for Healthcare Big Data Management and Analysis

Hao Gui[1], Rong Zheng[1], Chao Ma[1(✉)], Hao Fan[2], and Liya Xu[1]

[1] International School of Software, Wuhan University,
Wuhan, People's Republic of China
{hgui,rongz,chaoma,lyxu}@whu.edu.cn
[2] School of Information Management, Wuhan University,
Wuhan, People's Republic of China
hfan@whu.edu.cn

Abstract. Within the recent decades, data volume increases exponentially in different industries especially in healthcare field. Extracting the hidden value behind such massive data has become one of the hottest topics for both industry and academy. In this paper, we present an architecture for healthcare big data management and analysis. Under the guidance of the proposed architecture, a prototype system constructed based on HBase, Hive, Spark MLLib and Spark Streaming is introduced for personal health problem detection and real-time vital sign monitoring.

Keywords: Healthcare big data analysis · HBase · Hive · Spark MLLib · Spark Streaming

1 Introduction

Computer, Internet, big data, artificial intelligence, numerous emerging technologies are changing the world and almost every industry. In the healthcare field, more and more people are eager to conveniently obtain more intelligent healthcare services without seeing a doctor. For instance, a chronic disease patient is allowed to rest at home and he would like to know his body state which can be monitored by wearable medical devices. Such devices or systems are able to monitor patient's vital signs and send them to a remote data center. Both historical and realtime data can be utilized for further analysis and treatment suggestion. However, the amount of such data would be as large as we never saw before. We call it as healthcare big data with the following "5V" features.

- Volume: as estimated, by 2020, the healthcare data will dramatically increase to 35 ZBytes which is 43 times more than that in 2009.

This research is supported under the grant NO.71661167007 of National Natural Science of China.

X. Yin et al. (Eds.): HIS 2016, LNCS 10038, pp. 154–160, 2016.
DOI: 10.1007/978-3-319-48335-1_17

- Variety: healthcare data may be collected from multiple sources such as hospital information system, different medical sensors and with different formats such as structured, semi-structured, non-structured.
- Velocity: the healthcare data and domain knowledge in health field should be up to date.
- Veracity: the healthcare data should be provided by reputable healthcare agencies to guarantee data accuracy.
- Value: it is strongly believed that valuable information could be found by thoroughly analyzing healthcare big data.

However, no mater in theory or practice, the healthcare big data management and analysis is far from maturity. Hence, there are a lot of research issues and engineering challenges to tackle. In this paper, we present an architecture for healthcare big data management and analysis. Under the guidance of the proposed architecture, a prototype system constructed based on HBase, Hive, Spark MLLib and Spark Streaming is introduced for personal health problem detection and real-time vital sign monitoring.

The rest of this paper is organized as followed. In Sect. 2, the related works are discussed. In Sect. 3, the architecture for healthcare big data management and analysis is introduced with detailed illustration. In Sect. 4, a prototype system is described, built under the guidance of the proposed architecture to show its effectiveness. Finally, the conclusions and future works are provided.

2 Related Work

In [1], Wlodarczak and his partners described the techniques and algorithms used for reality mining and predictive analysis in eHealth Apps. They tried to make full use of the behavioral data from interactions from electronic exchanges (call records, email headers, SMS logs) and contextual data (location information) to detect deviations and alert care-takers based on predictive models.

In [2], Zhao and his teammates developed an automated method that is able to detect abnormal patterns of the elderly entering and exiting behaviors collected from simple sensors equipped in home-based setting. This method is based on Markov Chain Model and it can help classify abnormal sequences via analyzing the probability distribution of the spatiotemporal activity data.

In [3], Loper and his partners came up with a storage model that is based on Entity-Attribute-Value triples and this model is designed for health data in various formats. In this model, both the true and reference values are stored and it offers a very flexible approach to deal with different types of health data.

3 Architecture for Healthcare Big Data Analysis

The architecture proposed in this paper to tackle healthcare big data consists of five layers including Data Layer, Data Aggregation Layer, Analytics Layer, Information Exploration Layer, and Data Governance Layer. The proposed architecture is described in Fig. 1.

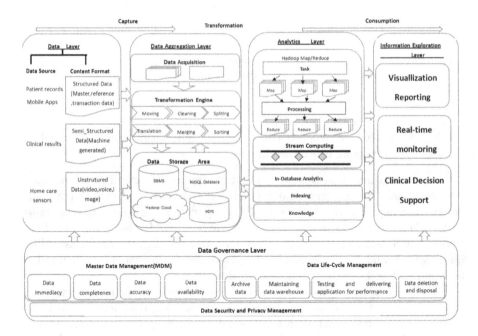

Fig. 1. Architecture for healthcare big data management and analysis

3.1 Data Layer

Healthcare data has multiple sources such as EHR (Electronic Health Record) and different types of medical devices. At the same time, the healthcare data is collected with different formats such as structured data, semi-structured data and unstructured data, which lead to the challenges for data collection and pre-processing.

The Data Layer of the proposed architecture aims to provide services facilitating data collection and pre-processing for popular HL7 compatible health records, back-end data of mobile healthcare Apps and streaming data generated by wearable medical sensors.

3.2 Data Aggregation Layer

The main tasks of the Data Aggregation Layer include data extraction, transformation and loading into storage system. With the support from Data Layer, necessary operations including data moving, cleaning, splitting, translation, merging, and sorting can be performed. Afterward, the healthcare big data with standard format can be loaded into a storage system which may be relational databases, NO-SQL databases, distributed file systems and etc.

3.3 Analytics Layer

With the support from the Data Aggregation Layer, the Analytic Layer focuses on basic statistical analysis work. Usually, work on this layer includes On-Line massive healthcare data analytical processing, streaming data processing, database construction & optimization, indexing, etc.

3.4 Information Exploration Layer

The Information Exploration Layer consists of visualization/reporting, real-time monitoring and clinical decision support. As we know, the healthcare big data could be massive and complex, which makes it difficult to understand and observe. Therefore, powerful techniques for efficiently visualizing and summarizing the healthcare big data become vital. And for patients, we care about analysis results on not only the historical data but also the current vital signs. For this purpose, real-time monitoring based on transient vital signs of patients is needed. Thanks to the recent development of big data technologies, there is a way to enable real-time monitoring by utilizing streaming-like techniques. Besides, according to the further investigation on historical clinical data, it is feasible to provide better clinical decision support for doctors. So far, some artificial intelligent algorithms such as Byesian model, logistic regression model, decision tree, support vector machine, random forest and others can be integrated with domain knowledge for clinical decision purposes.

3.5 Data Governance Layer

Data Governance Layer, which is integrated with all the other four layers, is responsible for meta-data management, data life-cycle management and security/privacy management.

4 Prototype System

Under the guidance of the proposed architecture, a prototype system is developed. The main function of the prototype system is to monitor blood pressure in a real-time manner and show warning information by comprehensively analyzing both historical and current blood pressure collected from patients.

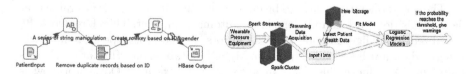

Fig. 2. Transformation in HBase

Fig. 3. Flowchart of Spark Streaming operations

On the Data Gathering Layer, a private cloud storage system is built with supports from VMWare virtualization technology. All the healthcare data are recorded in either HL7 [11] compatible EHR [12] documents (XML format) or the relational database MySQL.

For data aggregation purposes, Kettle [10] is utilized to conduct extraction, transformation, and loading operations on HL7 compatible documents while Sqoop [8] is chosen for conducting similar pre-processing operations on data stored in the MySQL database. Finally, healthcare data with different formats will be loaded into HBase [5] to support efficient query processing for operations on Data Analytic Layer. Firstly, patient XML-based records will be parsed by using XPath technique. Then, the rowkey will be constructed while raw data is pre-processed. After that, the duplicated records will be removed according to their IDs. A set of Javascripts enable the automatic generation of rowkeys. Finally, healthcare data with different formats can be loaded in to the HBase storage system. The flowchart of the above-mentioned process is described in Fig. 2. Furthermore, to make data loading successful in HBase, the mappings between data nodes and fields of HBase tables must be provided as shown in Fig. 4.

#	Alias	Key	Column family	Column name	Type	Indexed values
1	Rowkey	Y			String	
2	active	N	BasicInfo	ACT	String	
3	birthDate	N	BasicInfo	BD	String	
4	city	N	BasicInfo	C	String	
5	district	N	BasicInfo	D	String	
6	firstName	N	BasicInfo	FN	String	
7	gender	N	BasicInfo	G	String	
8	lastName	N	BasicInfo	LN	String	
9	line	N	BasicInfo	L	String	
10	postalCode	N	BasicInfo	PC	String	
11	reference	N	BasicInfo	reference	String	
12	state	N	BasicInfo	P	String	
13	telephone	N	BasicInfo	PN	String	

Configure connection | Create/Edit mappings

HBase table name: Person
Mapping name: PersonMapping

Fig. 4. Data mappings in HBase

UserID	Time	SDP	DBP
100	20160515212940	135	92
100	20160515212945	135	96
100	20160515212950	135	95
100	20160515212955	137	95
Warning:the probability has reached 0.6765!			
100	20160515213000	137	92
Warning:the probability has reached 0.6812!			
100	20160515213005	141	91
Warning:the probability has reached 0.6798!			
100	20160515213010	138	88
Warning:the probability has reached 0.6776!			
100	20160515213125	134	99

Fig. 5. Potential disease alarming UI

To complete ETL operations on the relational database while loading data into Hive [4], the first step is to design table structures in Hive. In the second step, relational database data will be loaded into Hive storage by registering the source database server address, account, password, and necessary drivers.

The above operations have to be done manually. However, it is desirable that data acquisition work can be done in an automatic manner. Therefore, Oozie [9] is utilized to configure Sqoop tasks as scripts. In the prototype system, newly generated data will be loaded from the MySQL database into Hive at everyday's midnight. To achieve this goal, an automatically executed Oozie workflow is defined which schedules the start-time, end-time, execution duration and other parameters of a Sqoop job for data loading purposes from MySQL to Hive.

So far, it is feasible to conveniently gather and aggregate healthcare big data into proper big data storage systems including HBase and Hive. We further hope that new important issues can be extracted from both static and dynamic healthcare data of patients. In the context of big data, dynamic data is also known as streaming data. In this prototype system, according to the healthcare domain knowledge, we aim to detect potential dangers of patients with elevated blood pressure by analyzing both their static information such as age, gender and dynamic data (i.e. instant blood pressure). Spark MLLib and Spark Streaming techniques are adopted for real-time blood pressure monitoring and on-line learning to decide wether the current state of patients is danger or not which is the supervised classification. The logistic regression model is selected for handling this supervised classification problem. The detailed data processing is shown in Fig. 3.

Finally, according to the historical data analysis in HBase, Hive and real-time blood pressure monitoring, the intelligent component (i.e. logistic regression model) of our prototype system is able to detect potential health problems of patients and give alarms like shown in Fig. 5.

5   Conclusions and Future Works

In this paper, an intelligent platform architecture for healthcare big data analysis is proposed for guiding the design and development of big data applications in the healthcare field. Under the guidance of the prosed architecture, a prototype system is developed in which HBase and Hive perform as storage components while Kettel and Sqoop are utilized for ETL operations. Finally, Spark Streaming and Spark MLLib are integrated into the prototype system for real-time monitoring and on-line decision support for patients with elevated blood pressure.

Since this is a prototype system, security and privacy issues are not considered. In the future, effective security and privacy techniques such as MD5 encryption and anonymity transformation would be integrated into the system. We will try more machine learning algorithms in Spark MLLib to tackle data mining tasks when facing big data in the healthcare field.

References

1. Wlodarczak, P., Soar, J., Ally, M.: Reality Mining in eHealth. In: Yin, X., Ho, K., Zeng, D., Aickelin, U., Zhou, R., Wang, H. (eds.) HIS 2015. LNCS, vol. 9085, pp. 1–6. Springer, Heidelberg (2015). doi:10.1007/978-3-319-19156-0_1
2. Zhao, T., Ni, H., Zhou, X., Qiang, L., Zhang, D., Yu, Z.: Detecting abnormal patterns of daily activities for the elderly living alone. In: Zhang, Y., Yao, G., He, J., Wang, L., Smalheiser, N.R., Yin, X. (eds.) HIS 2014. LNCS, vol. 8423, pp. 95–108. Springer, Heidelberg (2014). doi:10.1007/978-3-319-06269-3_11
3. Löper, D., Klettke, M., Bruder, I., Heuer, A.: Integrating healthcare-related information using the entity-attribute-value storage model. In: He, J., Liu, X., Krupinski, E.A., Xu, G. (eds.) HIS 2012. LNCS, vol. 7231, pp. 13–24. Springer, Heidelberg (2012). doi:10.1007/978-3-642-29361-0_4

4. Apache Hive. http://hive.apache.org
5. Apache HBase. http://hbase.apache.org
6. Apache Spark. http://spark.apache.org
7. Apache Hadoop. http://hadoop.apache.org
8. Apache Sqoop. http://sqoop.apache.org
9. Apache Oozie. http://oozie.apache.org
10. Kettle. http://community.pentaho.com/projects/data-integration
11. HL7. http://www.hl7.org
12. ERH. http://www.himss.org/library/ehr

Health Indicators Within EHR Systems in Primary Care Settings: Availability and Presentation

Xia Jing[1](✉), Francisca Lekey[1], Abigail Kacpura[2], and Kathy Jefford[2]

[1] The Department of Social and Public Health, College of Health Sciences and Professions, Ohio University, Athens, OH 45701, USA
jingx@ohio.edu
[2] Heritage College of Osteopathic Medicine, Ohio University, Athens, OH 45701, USA

Abstract. Prevention of disease, in addition to disease treatment, is recognized as an important component of a physician's role. High-quality prevention services can be used to detect diseases at an early stage, maintain the health of the population, and reduce healthcare costs. Precise and convenient measurement of the quality and delivery of prevention services, however, has not been adequately achieved. In this regard, primary care providers are the main workforce for the delivery of prevention services, and electronic health record (EHR) systems are the routine tools used for such delivery. In this paper, we review and summarize the currently used health indicators for measuring an individual's health status. We then visit and interview four primary care providers, who use four different EHR/EMR systems, to check the availability and presentation of these health indicators in these systems. We find that there are very limited health indicators available in *all* four systems. A re-examination of the EHR standards, to include more health indicators to measure prevention, is needed.

Keywords: Health indicators · Electronic Health Record Systems · General health status · Health status measurements · Primary care

1 Introduction

Electronic health record/electronic medical record (EHR/EMR) systems are a necessary and routine instrument for healthcare delivery. In the United States, by 2014, the adoption rates of EHR/EMR systems had reached 83 % [1] for physicians in general, 87 % [1] for primary care physicians, and over 94 % [2] for hospitals. When the focus of the healthcare shifts from treatment to prevention, primary care providers are one of the main workforces who provide delivery of preventive medicine services [3, 4]. There are, however, at least two challenges to delivering preventive medicine: (1) how to measure an individual's general health status objectively and accurately and (2) how to measure primary care providers' performance in delivering preventive medicine services. Accurate measurement is critical to improving prevention services delivery. In this paper, we first review the literature and summarize the health indicators that are used to measure an individual's health status. We then explore the availability and

© Springer International Publishing AG 2016
X. Yin et al. (Eds.): HIS 2016, LNCS 10038, pp. 161–167, 2016.
DOI: 10.1007/978-3-319-48335-1_18

presentation of the indicators in four convenience samples of EHR/EMR systems as well as providers' perceptions of existing preventive medicine panels within these EHR/EMR systems. To investigation of these health indicators and their availability in EHR systems is the first step of the project. Without capturing sufficient, consistent data, any further application and analysis of the data will be close to impossible.

The long-term goals are to capture preventive medicine services via EHR systems accurately, objectively, and conveniently as well as to measure individual's general health and providers' performance. The expected technical contribution of this project is to present the guidelines for and evidence of EHR development in regard to the core data elements and the value sets that should be included in a preventive medicine panel in an EHR system. EHR developers can implement the guideline by setting up tables within a database and utilizing the data elements and their value sets.

A set of health indicators is necessary because the indicators can be used to capture individuals' health status and to measure the performance of providers' preventive medicine services. Further, aggregated patients' health indicator data across institutions or over time (longitudinal) can be used to provide an overview of the health of the community (i.e., population level). The preventive medicine that we discuss in this paper concerns primary prevention (e.g., immunization, health-promotion activities, health consultations for smoking cessation), and secondary prevention (e.g., screening for diseases) [4].

2 Health Indicators: What are Being Used Now?

Health indicators refer to measurable items that can be used to demonstrate an *individual's* general health status, not a group's health status or even a disease's status. The health indicators for a group of people, such as mortality and morbidity, have been used for a long time as indicators of population health; this, however, is not the focus of this paper.

We examined the literature related to individual health indicators from peer-reviewed publications, official surveys (e.g., the National Health Interview Survey), and national rankings (e.g., American Health Rankings, Gallup Well-Being Index), and other reports. The inclusion criteria for the curated health indicators are (1) used for individuals, (2) used in primary care settings, (3) within the scope of primary prevention, (4) within the scope of secondary prevention, and (5) used before disease diagnosis. Exclusion criteria include (1) diseases-related indicators, (2) family-, community-, or population-related indicators, (3) health indicators within the scope of tertiary prevention, (4) health systems-related indicators, (5) indicators only for pregnancy, newborns, and children, and (6) indicators related to death. We summarize the individual health indicators in Table 1 [5–8]. We also included preventive medicine-related measurements in the Physician Quality Reporting System (PQRS) measurement list 2015 [9].

Table 1. Summary of current health indicators, measures, sources and availability

Health indicators	Current measures	No.
Health risks and behavior indicators [5]		
	Alcohol abuse* [5, 8, 9]	2/4
	Drug/substance abuse [5]	1/4
	Fruit/vegetable consumption [5, 9], diet and nutrition* [8]	¼
	Obesity/weight [5, 8], BMI* [7]	2/4
	Physical inactivity* [5, 8, 9]	1/4
	Smoking/tobacco use* [5, 8, 9]	2/4
	Sun protection [8]	
	Family history of cancer [8]	1/4
Healthcare [5]		
	Insurance coverage [5, 10]	
	Has a primary care provider* [10]	
	Immunization/vaccination* [5], influenza* [8], pneumococcal diseases* [8], hepatitis A [8], hepatitis B [8], tetanus [8], shingles [8], human papillomavirus [8]	4/4
	Unmet care needs [7]	
	Personal care needs [8]	
Health related quality of life (HRQL) [5]		
	Activity limitation [5]	
	Poor health days [5]	1/4
	Poor physical/mental health days [5]	
	Self-rated health status [5, 7, 8]	
High school diploma, recent drug use [5, 7, 9]		
Race ethnicity [5]		
Major depression* [5]		
	Preventable hospitalization [5]	
	Serious psychological distress [8]	1/4
Care provider supply [5]		
	Cancer screening/detection* [5, 8], colorectal cancer screening* [10]	4/4
	Hypertension screening* [5]	3/4
	Preventable hospitalization rate [7]	
	HIV testing* [8]	3/4
Dentist supply* [5, 10]		
Toxic chemicals/air quality standards [5, 10]		
	Air quality index > 100 [10]	
Unemployed individual [5]		

(Continued)

Table 1. (*Continued*)

Health indicators	Current measures	No.
Engaged people [7]		
	Health literacy rate [7]	
	Social support [7]	1/4
	Purpose [11]	1/4
Blood sugar level		4/4
Blood cholesterol		1/4
Blood triglycerides		1/4
HDL cholesterol		2/4
LDL cholesterol*		1/4

* = are listed in PQRS measurement list 2015; No. = availability of the health indicators in the four EHR/EMR systems.

3   Health Indicators in EHR/EMR Systems: Availability and Presentation

We visited four sites to collect data by observing and interviewing four primary care providers who use four different EHR/EMR systems (i.e., Amazing Charts, Athena-Health, Allscripts, and eClinicalWorks) in ambulatory settings. The providers include two physicians, one nurse practitioner, and one medical administrator. The availability of health indicators in the four EHR/EMR systems is summarized in Table 1.

The presentation of health indicators can be summarized as follows: (1) all four systems have preventive medicine panels; (2) all four systems have different health indicators available; (3) the health indicators are related to incentives in two systems; (4) two systems need to have health indicator data entered manually, and one system provides pre-defined lists; (5) two providers use the preventive medicine panel on a daily basis; (6) one provider thinks that the current health indicators are useful, another provider suggests that more health indicators of a complex lifestyle are needed, and a third provider thinks that, if the alerts are more automatic, then usage may be more frequent; (7) three providers would like to modify existing health indicators within the systems; and (8) three providers agree that primary care providers should record those indicators.

The four systems have different architectures, so the preventive medicine panel is different within each system: In two systems, the panel is under clinical decision support systems; in one, it is under health management plan, and, in the other, it is under quality management. Not all indicators, however, are listed only in the panel; some are captured in medical history, vital signs, social-economic data, or other categories.

4 Discussion

Although the value of prevention, as compared to treatment, has been recognized for a long time, only a limited portion of the population receives the corresponding prevention services. In the United States, by 2013, 41 % (adults aged 18 years and over who had received an influenza vaccination) to 70 % (children aged 19-35 months who had received the combined childhood vaccinations and women aged 18 and over who had a Pap smear in the past three years) of the population had received preventive medicine services [11, p25]. A personal health record (PHR) is believed to play an important role in the delivery of preventive medicine services. The low usage rate of PHRs, however, limits their full potential. Krist and colleagues developed a PHR [13], and their well-designed randomized trial [13–15] demonstrated that it can increase preventive medicine services delivery *if users adopt the PHR and use it*. In their studies, the PHR usage rate was 20 %. However, due to their high adoption and usage rate, EHR systems (87 % for primary care physicians [2]) can be a great platform to leverage delivery of preventive medicine services and to administer the services more effectively. According to U.S. national health statistics data [16], the volume of physician office visits (928.6 million in 2012) was about 7.4 times that of hospital visits (125.7 million in 2011). Further, 54.6 % of the physician office visits were made to primary care physicians. Primary care physicians are the main providers of preventive medicine services [3, 4]. In this regard, our long-term goal is to use EHR systems to capture preventive medicine services accurately, objectively, and conveniently. Thus, office-based practices are an appropriate setting from which to begin an investigation.

Whether current EHR/EMR systems have sufficient data elements to capture preventive medicine services is unknown. Because we investigated only four EHR/EMR systems, we must be cautious when attempting to generalize the results. According to our investigation, not all health indicators are included in the systems (Table 1). Further, if users are not familiar with the health indicator aspects of their systems, their results may not be accurate. Overall, we found that daily users are not able to locate *all* of the indicators instantly in any system.

The health indicators can be organized in other ways, e.g., categorization by diseases. The indicators will have to be validated and prioritized before they can be included in the EHR standards as core data elements and their value sets. Further, all corresponding data elements and value sets should follow controlled terminologies.

Some challenges needed to be addressed to achieve our long-term goal. The first challenge is to validate the health indicators. PQRS is used by the Centers for Medicare and Medicaid Services (CMS) to measure physicians' performance quality in the United States. There are 23 (9.02 %, 23/255) preventive medicine measures in the PQRS measure list 2015 [9]. Table 1 covers 78.26 % of these preventive medicine measures. In addition, a variety of professionals could validate the indicators. The second is to develop detailed and accurate guidelines that can be used to measure individual health precisely. For example, self-reported health status has been identified as the best current measure for well-being [7] (p. 135); however, the rating criteria for self-evaluation are unclear. The third is to prioritize the health indicators, and the fourth is to select the core data elements, without overwhelming the providers with information. Thus, future research should examine the health indicators of existing EHR standards, e.g., OpenEHR [17], clinical document architecture, the continuity of care document.

5 Conclusions

EHR/EMR systems can be used to capture individual health indicators and to accurately track the delivery of preventive medicine services. Very few health indicators, however, are captured in *all* four EHR/EMR systems investigated. To improve prevention services, we may need to re-examine the current EHR standards systematically to capture and measure preventive medicine services accurately.

Acknowledgements. Sincere thanks to all of the primary care providers participants as well as to Mr. Steve Davis, Dr. Douglas Bolon, Mr. Mark Bridenbaugh, and Ms. Tasha Penwell for helping us to connect with interviewees.

References

1. Heisey-Grove, D., Patel, V.: Any, Certified, or Basic: Quantifying Physician EHR Adoption. ONC Data Brief, no. 28. HealthIT.gov. 2015. http://dashboard.healthit.gov/evaluations/data-briefs/quantifying-physician-ehr-adoption.php
2. Office of the National Coordinator for Health Information Technology. Percent of Hospitals, By Type, that Possess Certified Health IT, Health IT Quick-Stat #52. HealthIT.gov. 2016. dashboard.healthit.gov/quickstats/pages/certified-electronic-health-record-technology-in-hospitals.php
3. Hensrud, D.: Clinical preventive medicine in primary care: background and practice: 1. Rationale and current preventive practices. Mayo Clin. Proc. **75**(2), 165–172 (2000). PMID: 10683656
4. Hensrud, D.: Clinical preventive medicine in primary care: background and practice: 2. delivering primary preventive services. Mayo Clin. Proc. **75**(3), 255–264 (2000). PMID: 10725952
5. Wold, C.: Health Indicators: a review of reports currently in use (2008). http://www.cherylwold.com/images/Wold_Indicators_July08.pdf
6. Committee on the State of the USA Health Indicators Institute of Medicine. State of the USA Health Indicators: Letter Report. The National Academies Press, Washington DC (2009)
7. Committee on core metrics for better health at lower cost: institute of medicine. In: Blumenthal, D., Malphrus, E., McGinnis, M. (eds.) Vital Signs: Core Metrics for Health and Health Care Progress, The National Academies Press, Washington DC (2015)
8. CDC. National Health Interview Survey. [cited 19 Feb 2016]. http://www.cdc.gov/nchs/nhis.htm
9. CMS. Physician quality reporting system (2015). https://www.cms.gov/Medicare/Quality-Initiatives-Patient-Assessment-Instruments/PQRS/index.html
10. Healthy People 2020 Leading Health Indicators: Progress Update (2014). http://www.healthypeople.gov/sites/default/files/LHI-ProgressReport-ExecSum_0.pdf
11. Gallup-Healthways Well-Being Index. State of global well-being: results of the Gallup-Healthways global well-being index (2014)

12. Statistics NC for H. Health, United States, 2014: with special feature on adults aged 55-64. Hyattsville, MD (2015). http://www.cdc.gov/nchs/data/hus/hus14.pdf#103
13. Krist, A., Peele, E., Woolf, S., Rothemich, S., Loomis, J., Longo, D., et al.: Designing a patient-centered personal health record to promote preventive care. BMC Med. Inf. Decis. Making **11**, 73 (2011)
14. Krist, A., Woolf, S., Rothemich, S., Johnson, R., Peele, J., Cunningham, T., et al.: Interactive preventive health record to enhance delivery of recommended care: a randomized trial. Ann. Fam. Med. **10**(4), 312–319 (2012)
15. Krist, A., Woolf, S.: A vision for patient-centered health informaiton systems. JAMA **305** (3), 300–301 (2011)
16. CDC. Ambulatory Care Use and Physician office visits (2014). http://www.cdc.gov/nchs/fastats/physician-visits.htm
17. OpenEHR. OpenEHR. http://www.openehr.org/

Statistical Modeling Adoption on the Late-Life Function and Disability Instrument Compared to Kansas City Cardiomyopathy Questionnaire

Yunkai Liu[✉] and A. Kate MacPhedran

Gannon University, Erie, PA, USA
{LIU006, MACPHEDRO01}@gannon.edu

Abstract. Transcatheter aortic valve replacement (TAVR) has become a more utilized procedure to perform on patients deemed too frail to handle the demands of a standard open heart approach. How to determine frailty in cardiac patients, particularly TAVR candidates, has been difficult to objectively quantify. The purpose of this research was to statistically measure which outcome tool most accurately depicted frailty in patients who underwent TAVR. Our study was performed based on the comparison between two approaches: the Kansas City Cardiomyopathy Questionnaire (KCCQ), which is the current national assessment standard conducted, and the Fried scale, which tests five frailty domains: gait speed, grip strength, low physical activity, exhaustion, and weight loss. Each domain of the Fried scale was explored and compared alongside the KCCQ with that frail/not frail to the TAVR patients with complications and deaths. Low physical activity was the strongest single-frailty domain predictor. Three statistical models – Logistic Regression, Support Vector Machines (SVM), and Artificial Neural Network (ANN), were used to build classification systems to predict complication conditions. Comparing static numbers, such as Sensitivity, Specificity and Area under Curve (AUC), it is believed that composed models based on the five domains of the Fried scale were able to demonstrate more accurate results than the traditional KCCQ approach. Both SVM and ANN showed significant performance, but further research is necessary to confirm specificity for the Fried scale with the TAVR population.

Keywords: Late-Life Function and Disability Instrument · Kansas City Cardiomyopathy Questionnaire · Fried's frailty phenotype · Logistic Regression · Artificial Neural Networks Model · Support Vector Machines

1 Introduction

The transcatheter aortic valve replacement (TAVR), was introduced in 2002 as an alternative, less invasive approach than traditional open sternotomy aortic valve replacement surgery, and intended specifically for individuals considered too "frail" to withstand traditional approach surgery [1, 2]. Research and advancing technology has since led to the emergence of the transapical and transaortic catheter approach in replacing the valve to further ameliorate the risk of morbidity and mortality in this high-risk patient population [1]. A potential candidate for TAVR is assessed through a

© Springer International Publishing AG 2016
X. Yin et al. (Eds.): HIS 2016, LNCS 10038, pp. 168–179, 2016.
DOI: 10.1007/978-3-319-48335-1_19

multi-disciplinary approach which is based predominantly on extensive cardiac testing, surgical feasibility and the various approaches [1, 3]. Surgeons also rely, in part, on a preoperative frailty assessment to help determine appropriateness for TAVR versus open approach and aid them in consideration of short and long-term postoperative survival [3, 4].

Frailty is multifactorial in nature and to date there has not been a universal definition agreed upon for this concept or a standardized method utilized to accurately identify who is frail [3, 5–7]. For this study, frailty is defined as a decline in physiological systems which are evident in one's physical functions and activities of daily living. The Kansas City Cardiomyopathy Questionnaire (KCCQ) is one of the most widely used health-related quality-of-life measures for patients with congestive heart failure [8, 9]. The KCCQ has been used in hundreds of clinical trials which have involved thousands of patients [8]. There is an inverse relationship between the KCCQ score and New York Heart Association (NYHA) classification, in that patients with low KCCQ scores indicate more advanced congestive heart failure symptoms and decreased quality of life [10, 11]. This valid and reliable tool is used to track progression of patients' conditions, when heart muscle has weakened due to prior heart attacks, heart valve problems, infections and the like, however, its symptoms section is specifically written for heart failure patients [5, 6].

With the KCCQs fairly strong correlation to the New York Heart Association Classifications [10, 11], this questionnaire has more recently been used to estimate functional status [9, 12, 13]. The 5-meter walk test and KCCQ are the standard "frailty" measures required by the national Transcatheter Valve Therapy (TVT) Registry for patients with severe aortic stenosis undergoing TAVR [6, 9, 14]. These tools are used to help estimate TAVR surgical risk and eligibility for the necessity of TAVR surgery, as well as help predict surgical outcomes and track postoperative progress [14–18]. Every TAVR candidate must have at least severe aortic stenosis, however, not every patient with severe aortic stenosis has cardiomyopathy and congestive heart failure [18, 19]. Thus, the KCCQ may fail to accurately capture frailty in this population.

Fried et al. proposed a different approach to assessing frailty, referred to clinically as the Fried scale, which is based on a frailty phenotype [7, 20]. The Fried scale's frailty phenotype is comprised of five domains: low physical activity, slow walk speed, unintended weight loss, exhaustion, and weak grip strength [7, 20]. Fried's frailty phenotype has been proven to be a valid frailty measurement and recognized as one the most commonly utilized measure of frailty [6, 16, 21].

The measurements for Fried's frailty scale are obtained through a combination of physiological tests and self-reported questionnaires [8]. To date, the frailty domain "low physical activity" has had wide variability in how it has been measured (E.g., Minnesota Leisure Time Activities Questionnaire; Katz Index of activities of daily living) [2, 3, 7, 20]. The Late-Life Function and Disability Instrument (LLFDI) is a well-established, valid and reliable outcome tool which calculates functional limitation and has been tested on 60 to 90 year olds and older adults with cardiovascular disease and status-post cardiac surgery, making the LLFDI an ideal tool to use for "low physical activity" measurement [22–26].

A brief description of each of the five frailty domains tested is listed as follows.

- Walk Speed – time to walk 15 feet at a comfortable pace. Abbreviated as "Gait" in this paper.
- Exhaustion – based on responses to questions about energy level and effort. Abbreviated as "Exha" in this paper.
- Weight Loss – unintentional weight loss ($\geq 10\#$ in the last 12 months); answered as yes/no. Abbreviated as "WeLoss" in this paper.
- Grip Strength – measured using a hand-held dynamometer squeezed with the dominant hand. Abbreviated as "Grip" in this paper.
- Low Physical Activity – based on routine physical activities and daily tasks using the function component of the LLFDI [22]. Abbreviated as "LPA" in this paper.

The purpose of this study was to determine the predictive power of two different measurement tools in depicting frailty in patients with severe aortic stenosis who undergo TAVR. Every domain of the Fried scale is explored in detail and compared against the KCCQ with respect to patient complications and deaths. Three statistical models – Logistic Regression, Support Vector Machines (SVM), and Neural Network, were utilized to build classification systems in order to predict complication conditions. Comparing static numbers such as Sensitivity, Specificity and Area under Curve (AUC), it is believed that composed models based on the five domains of Fried's frailty scale are able to demonstrate more accurate results than the traditional KCCQ approach.

2   Data Collection

A retrospective cohort design was used to assess frailty data on 70 high-risk patients who were referred to Saint Vincent Hospital's multi-disciplinary TAVR team for possible TAVR procedure, between April, 2013 and October, 2014. Patients who were under 65 years, did not communicate fluently in English, or ended up not undergoing TAVR surgery for any reason (25 of the 70 referrals), were excluded from the study. Informed consent was originally obtained on all 70 patients to participate in the TAVR work-up process which included undergoing a preoperative frailty assessment. Institutional Review Board approval was obtained from both Saint Vincent Hospital and Gannon University, as this was a collaborative venture. All individual patient information was de-identified before any analysis conducted.

Frailty assessment measurements were based on the frailty phenotype operationalized by Fried et al. [7, 20] which is made up of slow gait speed, weak grip strength, shrinkage (weight loss), exhaustion, and low physical activity. Patients with impairments in at least three of the five domains were considered frail. Each patient had grip strength measured (average of 3 trials in kg) using a Jaymar dynamometer and patients whose average scores were in the lowest 20 % of community older adults, as based on gender and body mass index (on average: <30 kg for men, <19 kg for women), met criteria as having weak grip strength. Five meter walk speed was calculated (average of 3 trials) with patients cued to walk at a comfortable pace with or without a device. Gait speeds in the lowest 20 % of community older adults as based on sex and height cut-offs (either >6 or 7 s) met criteria for slow gait. Patients also answered 32 standardized questions on routine physical activities and daily tasks using the LLFDI, which asks "How much difficulty do you have...?" on a 1–5 Likert scale which was then converted to 0–100 point weighted scale, with a lower scale indicating increased limitation in physical mobility and activities of daily living, with a cut-off score at 52.5. Exhaustion was assessed according to self-report, using two standardized questions obtained from the Center for Epidemiologic Studies Depression Scale: "How often in the last week did you feel (1) everything was an effort; (2) you could not get going?" Answering either question as "3 or more days of the week" was considered "low endurance/exhausted," and met criteria. Unintentional weight loss of 10 or more pounds within the last year was self-reported and anyone noting such was considered having met the criterion for shrinkage/impaired nutrition.

Patients were also assessed according to the KCCQ which is a 12 question self-report on their physical function, congestive heart failure symptoms, quality of life, and social limitations [9]. The KCCQ is on a 1–5 or 1–7 Likert scale (depending on the question) which is converted to 0–100 summary score [9].

Baseline demographic information as well as all-cause mortality and complications which occurred up to 30 days postoperatively were assessed retrospectively via chart reviews. Postoperative complications included major bleeding, minor vascular, major vascular, stroke, new arrhythmia (requiring pacemaker), and acute renal injury, which are the reportable complications per TVT Registry criteria [27]. Verification of chart information (E.g., corrective vascular procedures) was confirmed by TAVR team members and all-cause mortality at 30 days was assessed per follow-up visit notes or phone calls (if visits were missed) by TAVR team members.

Table 1. Patient data demographics vs. TVT registry data

Patient Data (% or mean)	TVT Registry Data (% or mean)
n = **45** (from 04/13–10/14)	n = **12,182** (from11/11–06/13)
Age 81.5 (60–95 range)	Age 84 (79–88 range)
Female 22 (48.9 %)	Female n = 6,316 (51.9 %)
Caucasian 45 (100 %)	Caucasian n = 11, 615 (95.3 %)
TIA or Stroke 9 (20 %)	Chronic CHF 36 (80 %)
Cancer 8 (17.8 %)	30 day mortality = 7 %
Chronic renal failure 18 (40 %)	**PARTNER Trial Data**[a] **(n = 348)**
Stroke at 30 days 2 (4.4 %)	30 day stroke incidence = [a]4.1 %
Arrhythmia 3 (6.7 %)	Pacemaker needed = [a]6.4 %
Bleeding 2 (4.4 %)	Bleeding = [a]15.7 %
Minor vascular 4 (8.9 %)	Minor vascular = n/a
Major vascular 1 (2.2 %)	Major and minor vascular = [a]11.3 %
NYHA class III/IV 43 (95.6 %)	NYHA class III/IV = [a]94.3 %
30-Day mortality 3 (6.7 %)	30 day mortality = [b]5 %
30-Day complications 12 (26.7 %)	

TIA = Transient Ischemic Attack; CHF = Congestive Heart Failure
NYHA = New York Heart Association (Classifications);
TVT = Transcatheter Valve Therapy (Registry)
[a] PARTNER Trial = National study using TVT Registry to estimate risks
[b] = mortality rate was based on high-risk TAVR patients

3 Results - Baseline Demographics

Descriptive analysis from chart reviews were conducted on those identified as frail and on the entire sample, to compare to the surgical population as a whole. Baseline demographics (see Table 1) revealed that the study population was comprised entirely of Caucasian individuals, ranging in age from 60 to 95 (mean was 81.5) and females made up 48.9 %. Base on the data of those that underwent TAVR (n = 45), at 30 days postoperatively, a total of 2 patients (4.4 %) had suffered a stroke, 2 patients had bleeding issues, and 5 patients (11.1 %) had vascular issues, either minor or major, with the latter requiring surgical repair. Thirty-day complications overall were noted in 12 patients (26.7 %) and the mortality rate at 30-days was 6.7 % (3 patients).

4 Each Domain of the Fried Scale

Terms in Fig. 1 and related static values are listed as follows.

- Gait is the score of gait domain. The range was from 0 to 30 (seconds). The higher score means slower gait speed with frail cut-off at/above 6 s. In our dataset, the mean was 10.52 s and the median was 8.77 s.
- Exha is the score of exhaustion domain. The range is from 0 to 3 (Likert scale), with 0 is the best condition, and 3 is the worst condition. In our dataset, the mean was 2.16 and the median was 3.00.
- WeLoss is the score of weight loss domain. 0 means negative for unexpected weight loss, and 1 means positive. In our dataset, the mean was 0.42 and the median was 0.00.
- Grip is the score of grip domain. The range was from 0 to 50 (kg). The higher score means lower grip strength with gross cut-off <30 kg (for men) and <19 kg (for women) as frail. In our dataset, the mean was 12.95 and the median was 13.67.
- LPA is the score of low physical activity domain. The range was from 0 to 100 (converted LLFDI raw scale). In our dataset, the mean was 37.89 and the median was 43.44. The mean fell in the "severe limitation" category and median fell in the "moderate to severe limitation" category.
- Resp is a Boolean value to demonstrate complication or death status. 0 means patients without complication or death, and 1 means otherwise.

Figure 1 demonstrated some relationship of complications or deaths with each domain. For example, when Resp equals 1, most LPA data are in the range from 40 to 50; when Resp equals 0, most Gait data are in the range from 5 to 15. In addition, the relationship among five domains can be noticed. For instance, when Exha equals 3, most LPA data are in the range from 40 to 50, which means most patients with exhaustion have low physical activities.

Contingency tables were constructed to calculate negative and positive predictor values for frailty and the sensitivity and specificity of each measurement tool. The cohort was dichotomized into 2 groups "with complications or death within 30 days" versus "no complications or death within 30 days."

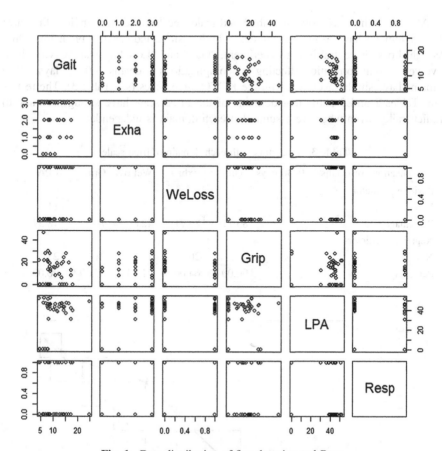

Fig. 1. Data distribution of five domains and Resp

Table 2. Predictive power of KCCQ

KCCQ Score 45–100 (Not Frail) vs. KCCQ Score 0–44 (Frail)	
True positive (TP) = 12 **False positive (FP) = 27**	**Positive predictive value** = TP/(TP + FP) = 12/(12 + 27) = 30.77 %
True negative (TN) = 4 **False negative (FN) = 2**	**Negative predictive value** = TN/(FN + TN) = 4/(2 + 4) = 67.77 %
Sensitivity **= TP/(TP + FN)** =12/(12 + 2) = 85.7 %	**Specificity** = TN/(FP + TN) = 4/(27 + 4) = 12.9 %

After exploring each domain of the Fried scale (see Table 2), it is obvious that most of the 5 domains have strong correlations as both positive and negative predictors. Only "Weight Loss" is neutral in our experiment. "Gait" and "Low Physical Activity" both have very strong correlation affecting to "complications or deaths in 0–30 days." Two domains have similar accuracy with the KCCQ approaches (see Table 3). The results from Tables 2 and 3 show that domains of the Fried scale have strong accuracy to predict frailty, even when we assume that each domain is independent.

Table 3. Predictors with each domain of fried scale

Complications or deaths in 0–30 days	Gait	Exha	WeLoss	Grip	LPA
Positive predictors					
N = 14	12	12	6	11	11
Percentage	85.71 %	85.71 %	42.86 %	78.57 %	78.57 %
Negative predictors					
N = 31	28	20	13	21	28
Percentage	90.00 %	64.00 %	41.00 %	67.00 %	90.00 %

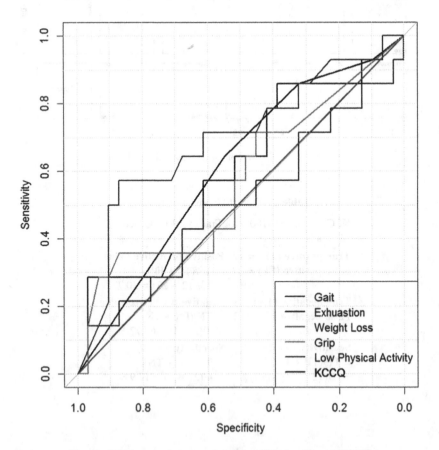

Fig. 2. ROC curves between domains of fried scale and KCCQ

Table 4. AUC values between domains of fried scale and KCCQ

Gait	Exha	WeLoss	Grip	LPA	KCCQ
0.5023	0.6094	0.5046	0.5703	0.6947	0.6025

Receiver operating characteristic (ROC) curves were computed to determine the predictive accuracy in identifying frailty, as those who truly had complications or death within 30 days. The ROC curves between five domains of the Fried scale and KCCQ are demonstrated in Fig. 2. Area under the ROC curve (AUC) was computed for each of Fried's frailty domains, the composite frailty phenotype (including the LLFDI scale), and the KCCQ and dichotomous cut points for predicting frailty were determined based on optimal crossing for sensitivity and specificity.

Based on results of Fig. 2 and Table 4, it is easy to conclude that "Low Physical Activity" is the most important and accurate domain of the Fried scale. Furthermore, KCCQ does not have strong accuracy and high AUC numbers, even though it is a popular approach.

5   Classify Domains of Fried Scale Using Three Statistical Models

In this section, three different statistical models are applied to classify the domains of the Fried scale. The purpose is to find a better mathematical model to predict frail. A comparison with the KCCQ approach is also studied. All calculations are performed under R environments. Several R packages, such as General Linear Modeling, SVM and neural network model are applied in the research. And the major measurements to evaluate those three methods are specificity, sensitivity, and AUC.

Some conclusions are drawn based on the comparison results from Fig. 3 and Table 5.

- KCCQ classification system has lower specificity, sensitivity and AUC. It is only similar with simple approach, such as logistic regression.
- SVM has the higher performance in specificity, sensitivity and AUC. Neural network model also shows relatively high performance.

The study shows the feasibility to use statistical model to predict frail based on domains of the Fried scale.

Table 5. Specificity, sensitivity, AUC of KCCQ classification system, logistic regression model, SVM model and neural network model

	KCCQ classification system	Logistic regression model	SVM model	Neural network model
Specificity	62 %	81 %	91 %	86 %
Sensitivity	59 %	58 %	92 %	81 %
AUC	0.6025	0.6682	0.9286	0.8986

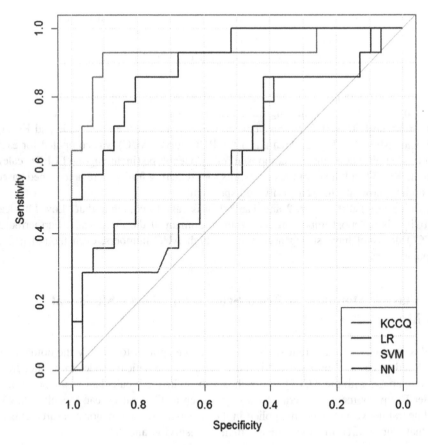

Fig. 3. ROC curves of KCCQ classification system, logistic regression model, SVM model and neural network model

6   Conclusions and Discussion

First off, patient characteristics of the study revealed that our demographics were a classic representation of what has been seen in the literature with TAVR patients [10, 16, 27]. Among our sample as well as patients undergoing TAVR in the U.S., both comprised similar demographics in gender make-up, mean age, and ethnicity [10, 16, 27]. Also similar in findings were the incidence of postoperative complications, both in our sample and the national TVT Registry data, examining 30-day incidence of stroke, vascular complications and overall mortality rate [16, 27]. Despite the data being obtained from a single center, the sample appears to well represent the general population of TAVR patients as a whole.

In this research paper, domains of the Fried scale were carefully explored. Based on our result, traditional KCCQ approach only show neutral accuracy. KCCQ and individual domains of the Fried scale have high sensitivity in detecting "truly frail." Among five domains, "Low Physical Activity," as measured by the LLFDI, appears to be the strongest single-frailty phenotype predictor. Exhaustion and grip strength also act as strong predictors of postoperative complications. Furthermore, three different statistical models are applied to integrate domains of the Fried scale. SVM model shows the most impressive performance based on specificity, sensitivity and AUC. Artificial neural network model also shows higher performance than the KCCQ approach.

However, the study is still preliminary. This sample had numerous comorbidities preoperatively, and in terms of TAVR surgical outcomes, this certainly could have impacted the findings. These patients were part of the first year this TAVR program was in practice, hence, there is a learning curve for any TAVR team, and until the experience levels and skill sets of the doctors and surgeons improve over time, this can also negatively impact postoperative complications, as has been documented in research and now appearing in national guidelines [2, 27, 28].

In the future, researchers may want to conduct repeated measures of the Fried scale postoperatively, beyond the initial preoperative frailty data, to calculate hazard ratios in order to determine survival trends between those that had complications versus no complications. There was difficulty with a small dataset to generalize findings and for such a reason, we suspect the Artificial Neural Network model may provide more convincing results with a bigger dataset. Furthermore, with a small sample, we were unable to dichotomize groups between frail and not frail to explore further nuances.

References

1. Alfirevic, A., Mehta, A.R., Svensson, L.G.: Trans catheter aortic valve replacement. Anesthesiol. Clin. **31**, 355–381 (2013)
2. Puls, M., Sobisiak, B., Bleckmann, A., et al.: Impact of frailty on short- and long-term morbidity and mortality after transcatheter aortic valve implantation: risk assessment by Katz Index of activities of daily living. EuroIntervention **10**, 609–619 (2014)
3. Afilalo, J., Alexander, K., Mack, M., et al.: Frailty assessment in the cardiovascular care of older adults. J. Am. Coll. Cardiol. **63**, 747–762 (2014)
4. Bagnall, N., Faiz, O., Darzi, A., et al.: What is the utility of preoperative frailty assessment for risk stratification in cardiac surgery? Interact. Cardiovasc. Thoarc. Surg. **14**, 398–402 (2013)
5. de Vries, N.M., Staal, J.B., van Ravensberg, C.D., et al.: Outcome instruments to measure frailty: a systematic review. Ageing Res. Rev. **10**, 104–114 (2010)
6. Mack, M.: Frailty and aortic valve disease. J. Cardiovasc. Surg. **145**, S7–10 (2013)
7. Makary, M., Segev, D., Pronovost, P., et al.: Frailty as a predictor of surgical outcomes in older patients. J. Am. Coll. Surg. **210**, 901–908 (2010)
8. Garin, O., Ferrer, M., Pont, A., et al.: Disease-specific health-related quality of life questionnaires for heart failure: a systematic review with meta-analyses. Qual. Life Res. **18**, 71–85 (2009)
9. Green, C., Porter, C., Bresnaham, D., et al.: Development and evaluation of the Kansas City Cardiomyopathy Questionnaire: a new health status measure for heart failure. J. Am. Coll. Cardiol. **35**, 1245–1255 (2000)

10. Reynolds, M., Magnuson, E., Wang, K., et al.: Health-related quality of life after transcatheter or surgical aortic valve replacement in high-risk patients with severe aortic stenosis: results from the PARTNER (Placement of AoRTic TraNscathetER Valve) Trial (cohort A). J. Am. Coll. Cardiol. **60**, 548–558 (2012)

11. Spertus, J., Peterson, E., Conard, M.W., et al.: Monitoring clinical changes in patients with heart failure: a comparison of methods. Am. Heart J. **150**, 707–715 (2005)

12. Schoenenberger, A.W., Stortecky, S., Neumann, S., et al.: Predictors of functional decline in elderly patients undergoing transcatheter aortic valve implantation (TAVI). Eur. Heart J. (2012). Epub ahead of print

13. Arnold, S., Spertus, J., Lei, Y., et al.: Use of the Kansas City Cardiomyopathy Questionnaire for monitoring health status in patients with aortic stenosis. Cir. Heart Fail. **6**, 61–67 (2013)

14. Afilalo, J., Eisenberg, M., Morin, J.F., et al.: Gait speed as an incremental predictor of mortality and major morbidity in elderly patients undergoing cardiac surgery. J. Am. Coll. Cardiol. **56**(20), 1668–1676 (2010)

15. Green, P.: Defining and measuring frailty: an important assessment feature of high risk TAVR patients. J. Am. Coll. Cardiol. Intv. **5**, 974 (2012)

16. Green, P., Woglom, A.E., Genereux, P., et al.: The impact of frailty status on survival after transcatheter aortic valve replacement in older adults with severe aortic stenosis. J. Am. Coll. Cardiol. Intv. **5**, 974–981 (2012)

17. Wilson, C.M., Kostsuca, S.R.K., Boura, J.A.: Utilization of a 5-Meter Walk Test in evaluating self-selected gait speed during preoperative screening of patients scheduled for cardiac surgery. Cardiopulm. Phys. Ther. J. **24**, 36–43 (2013)

18. Bean, J.F., Olveczky, D.D., Kiely, D.K., et al.: Performance-based versus patient-reported physical function: what are the underlying predictors? Phys. Ther. **91**, 1804–1811 (2011)

19. Dineen, E., Brent, B.: Aortic valve stenosis: comparison of patient with to those without chronic congestive heart failure. Am. J. Cardiol. **57**, 419–422 (1986)

20. Fried, L.P., Tangen, C.M., Walston, J., et al.: Frailty in older adults: evidence for a phenotype. J. Gerontol. **56**, 146–156 (2000)

21. Bouillon, K., Kivimaki, M., Hamer, M., et al.: Measures of frailty in population based studies: an overview. BMC Geriatr. **13**(64), 2–11 (2013)

22. Haley, S.M., Jette, A.M., Coster, W.J., et al.: Late life function and disability instrument: II. development and evaluation of the function component. J. Gerontol. Med. Sci. **57A**, M217–M222 (2002)

23. Kinney LaPier, T.K., Mizner, R.: Outcome measures in cardiopulmonary physical therapy: focus on the late life function and disability instrument (LLFDI). Cardiopulm. Phys. Ther. J. **20**(2), 32–35 (2009)

24. Kinney, T.K.: LaPier: utility of the late life function and disability instrument as an outcome measure in patients participating in outpatient cardiac rehabilitation: a preliminary study. Physiother. Can. **64**(1), 53–62 (2012)

25. Sayers, S.P., Jette, A.M., Haley, S.M., et al.: Validation of the late-life function and disability instrument. J. Am. Geriatr. Soc. **52**, 1554–1559 (2004)

26. Dubuc, N., Haley, S.M., Ni, P., et al.: Function and disability in late life: comparision of the late-life function and disability instrument to the short-form-36 and the London handicap scale. Disabil. Rehabil. **26**, 362–370 (2004)

27. Holmes, D.R., Mack, M.J., Kaul, S., et al.: ACCF/ AATS/SCAI/STS expert consensus document on transcatheter aortic valve replacement. J. Am. Coll. Cardiol. **59**(13), 1200–1254 (2012)

28. Osnabrugge, R.L.J., Mylotte, D., Head, S.J., et al.: Aortic stenosis in the elderly-disease prevalence and number of candidates for transcatheter aortic valve replacement: a meta-analysis and modeling study. J. Am. Coll. Cardiol. **62**(11), 1002–1012 (2013)

29. Vapnik, V.N., Vapnik, V.: Statistical Learning Theory. Wiley, New York (1998)
30. Dobson, A.J.: An Introduction to Generalized Linear Models. Chapman and Hall, London (1990)
31. Venables, W.N., Ripley, B.D.: Modern Applied Statistics with S. Springer, New York (2002)
32. Bennett, K.P., Campbell, C.: Support vector machines: hype or Hallelujah? SIGKDD Explor. 2(2) (2000)
33. Cortes, C., Vapnik, V.: Support-vector network. Mach. Learn. 20, 1–25 (1995)
34. Murata, et al.: Network information criterion determining the number of hidden units for an artificial neural network model. IEEE Trans. Neural Netw. 5(6), 865–871 (1994)
35. Anastasiadis, A., et al.: New globally convergent training scheme based on the resilient propagation algorithm. Neurocomputing 64, 253–270 (2005)

A Case Study on Epidemic Disease Cartography Using Geographic Information

Changbin Yu[1,2(✉)], Jiangang Yang[3], Yiwen Wang[1,2], Ke Huang[1,2],
Honglei Cui[1,2], Mingfang Dai[4], Hongjian Chen[5], Yu Liu[6],
and Zhensheng Wang[7]

[1] Sino-Aus Research Center on Social Computing and Data Management,
Ningbo Institute of Technology, Zhejiang University, No. 1 Xuefu Road,
Ningbo 315010, Zhejiang, China
{240212388,1293024839,9259536,2814107537}@qq.com
[2] School of Management, Ningbo Institute of Technology, Zhejiang University,
No. 1 Xuefu Road, Ningbo 315010, Zhejiang, China
[3] College of Computer Science and Technology, Zhejiang University,
No. 866 Yuhangtang Road, Xihu District, Hangzhou 310058, Zhejiang, China
yangjg@cs.zju.edu.cn
[4] Ningbo Zhongjing Technology Development Limited Cooperation,
Ningbo 315010, Zhejiang, China
18787706@qq.com
[5] Ningbo Yizhou Institute of Surveying and Mapping,
Ningbo 315010, Zhejiang, China
pmaster.cn@gmail.com
[6] Service Center for Registration of Immovables in Ningbo,
Ningbo 315010, Zhejiang, China
277936238@qq.com
[7] Shenzhen Key Laboratory of Spatial Information Smart Sensing and Services,
Shenzhen 518060, China
wangzhensheng@szu.edu.cn

Abstract. Research of epidemiology is one of the important components in the field of public health while spatial epidemiology combing traditional epidemiology with Geographic Information Science is often regarded as an effective way for visualization analysis. Here we conduct a disease study under the help of spatial technologies using one-year real epidemic data collected from Ningbo, Zhejiang, China where an epidemic cartography approach taking data scale into account is newly proposed and elaborated. The demonstrated experimental results indicate that the proposed method performs more flexible for analysis than that of traditional statistical methods.

Keywords: Geographic information science · Spatial epidemiology · Disease mapping · Data scale

© Springer International Publishing AG 2016
X. Yin et al. (Eds.): HIS 2016, LNCS 10038, pp. 180–193, 2016.
DOI: 10.1007/978-3-319-48335-1_20

1   Introduction

Closely related to our life quality, epidemiology is an important component in the field of public health and smarter health-care. Spatial epidemiology is a discipline that studies traditional epidemiology using the knowledge of geographic information science (GIS). It has been widely used to visually express the geographic locations and variations of epidemic diseases in terms of demographic, environments, genetics, and infectious risk factors, etc. [4, 10–12, 16, 22, 29]. A well-known application example of spatial epidemiology was the successful investigation of a cholera outbreak caused by street water pump pollution in London in 1854.

Since the core research of GIS is on spatial analysis and cartography [5, 6, 27], spatial epidemiology mainly focuses on four aspects including (1) spatial clustering analysis [1, 3, 9, 15, 25], (2) spatial auto-correlation analysis [2], (3) simulation of disease spreading process [14, 24] and (4) disease cartography [7, 8, 13, 17–19, 21, 23] (especially thematic cartography for disease visualization [26–28]). It should be noticed that, disease cartography has the ability to visually present the results of spatial clustering analysis, spatial auto-correlation analysis and simulation of disease spreading process, so disease cartography is emphasized on here.

Furthermore, current approaches and methods on epidemiology cartography mainly depend on categorical or numerical values. In detail, 'Quick Plot' is a valuable tool for visualization of categorical variables in epidemiological data [20] while SOM (Self-organizing Map) is also suitable [10]. Simple thematic mapping approaches (typically graded thematic mapping) is employed for numerical indicators describing diseases in different administrative regions [16] where interpolation methods such as kriging interpolation could also be applied to numerical values [8]. After reviewing related research, it can be found that, up to now, not a cartography approach for diseases taking data scale into account has been proposed yet. There, we will focus on disease cartography here and the study done here has the following contributions:

– From the perspective of theory, different from traditional thematic cartography for epidemiology, a cartography approach taking data scale including nominal scale, sequence scale, interval scale and ratio scale into consideration is newly proposed here.
– From the perspective of practice, we conducted a disease cartography study using real epidemic data of Ningbo city and provided thematic cartography on parameters such as spatial locations, age, gender, profession of infected individuals. The visualized results suggested a better understanding on the clustering of infectious diseases and estimation of influencing factors for each type of infectious disease which could be hardly achieved through traditional statistical based approaches.
– The demonstrated experimental results could be used to help the policy maker to conduct a correct policy for the diseases control.

   The rest of the paper is organized as follows. Section 2 illustrates the role of GIS in spatial epidemiology. Section 3 details the thematic cartography for epidemiology especially taking data scale into consideration. Section 4 is the actual case study for Ningbo city. Section 5 concludes this paper where clinical significance from analysis is also involved.

2 The Role of GIS in Spatial Epidemiology

Four tightly associated aspects in the field of spatial epidemiology are elaborated here including: (i) spatial clustering analysis, (ii) spatial correlation analysis (also called spatial auto-correlation analysis), (iii) simulation of disease spreading process (also called design of disease propagation model) and (iv) disease mapping or cartography (especially thematic cartography for disease). As mentioned above, the first three points (i)–(iii) are the foundation of the fourth point (iv), so the first three points are briefly reviewed in this section firstly, and then the fourth point will be elaborated in the next section.

2.1 Spatial Cluster

Generally, in the traditional field of computer science, 'cluster analysis' groups data objects into clusters such that objects belonging to the same cluster are similar, while those belonging to different ones are dissimilar. Based on the above, 'spatial cluster analysis' extends 'cluster analysis' in the domain of space which could be viewed intuitively. And cluster results are beneficial to find 'hot regions (hot spots)' or 'cold regions (cold spots)' for distribution of epidemiology. Approaches (or algorithms) for cluster analysis are usually categorized as follows: (i) partitional approaches including k-means algorithm; (ii) hierarchical approaches: including BIRCH algorithm; (iii) density-based approaches including DBSCAN algorithm; (iv) grid-based approaches including CLIQUE algorithm and (v) model-based approaches including COB-WEB algorithm.

2.2 Spatial Auto-correlation

As one of the most essential principles in the field of Geography, "the First Law in Geography" says: More Closer when two things are in the measure of Spatial Distances, More Related they are in the Measure of Association. This phenomenon is often regarded as "spatial auto-correlation" (also termed as "spatial auto-association"). Furthermore, it could be categorized into following: (i) positive correlation where high (or low) values are spatially surrounded by high (or low) values, (ii) negative correlation where high (or low) values are spatially surrounded by low (or high) values, and (iii) none correlation where no significant spatially surrounding trend is found.

In fact, it exist many indexes to answer the questions about spatial aggregation or spatial clustering, e.g. Moran' I indicator (including global ones and local ones), Getis-Ord indicator (including global ones and local ones), spatial statistic indicators, Geary' C indicator, Moran scatter plots, etc. These indexes playing important roles in exploration data analysis (especially in exploratory spatial data analysis) have distinguished characteristics where calculation of two indexes (global and local Moran' I indicators) is given here.

In detail, global Moran' I index is calculated using Eqs. (1) and (2):

$$I = \frac{\sum_{i=1}^{n}\sum_{j=1}^{n} w_{ij}(x_i - \bar{x})(x_j - \bar{x})}{S^2 * \sum_{i=1}^{n}\sum_{j=1}^{n} w_{ij}} (i \neq j) \tag{1}$$

$$S^2 = \frac{1}{n}\sum_{i=1}^{n}(x_i - \bar{x})^2, \quad \bar{x} = \frac{1}{n}\sum_{i=1}^{n} x_i \tag{2}$$

In Eq. (1), n denotes the number of samples, x_i and x_j denote the attribute value of i point and j point respectively. And w_{ij} denotes the weight measuring spatial relationships, i.e., when points are adjacent, w_{ij} equals 1; otherwise, w_{ij} equals 0. So, nominator of global Moran' I indicator ranges from -1 to $+1$ where $+1$ shows positive association, -1 shows negative association and 0 shows no association. Besides these, Eq. (2) explains how the denominator of global Moran' I indicator is calculated while calculation of the average value for attribute x is also explained.

In addition, local Moran' I index is calculated using Eqs. (3) and (4) where variables are similarly defined:

$$I_i = \frac{(x_i - \bar{x})}{S^2} \sum_{j=1}^{n} w_{ij}(x_j - \bar{x}) \tag{3}$$

$$S^2 = \frac{\sum_{j=1, j \neq i}^{n} w_{ij}(x_j - \bar{x})^2}{n - 1} \tag{4}$$

2.3 Simulation of Disease Spreading Process

Results of spatial cluster analysis using cluster algorithms and results of spatial auto-correlation analysis using auto-correlation indexes could be regarded as statistic results. By contrast, simulation of dynamic process for current epidemiology spreading is also necessary for further prediction of disease diffusion. Typical models for simulation of disease spreading cover SIS (Susceptible-Infective-Susceptible) model, SIR (Susceptible-Infective-Recovery) model, SEIR (Susceptible-Exposed-Infective-Recovery) model and SEIRW (Susceptible-Exposed-Infective-Recovered-Immune) model. These models emphasize on numerical calculation of spreading process taking factors including susceptible individuals, infective individuals, recovering individuals into account where dynamic process could not be viewed intuitively. By contrast, spatial models could also be employed for simulation of disease spreading. Cellular Automata Model is a typical spatial model where gradual spreading could be directly reflected in the domain of space.

3   Thematic Cartography for Epidemiology

Disease cartography (also called disease mapping) could be employed not only (i) as traditional final presentation results of cluster analysis output, spatial auto-correlation output and spreading process output, but also (ii) as a new visualization approach for further analysis using mapping especially thematic cartography.

For the former (i), lots of thematic cartographic approaches could be used, such as pyramid map, regional statistical map, positioning map and table, point-symbol, etc. where approaches are suitable for different situations (e.g., a single attribute/multiple attributes, a single year/multiple years) as elaborated in Fig. 1.

Representing Approaches	Statistical Attributes of Thematic Maps				
	Spatial location	A Single Indicator	Multiple Indicators	A Single Year	Multiple Years
Graduated statistical map	*Statistical region*	*Yes*	*No*	*Yes*	*No*
Pyramid map	*Statistical region and locating point*	*Yes*	*Yes (usually 2 indicators)*	*Yes*	*No*
Regional statistical map	*Statistical region*	*Yes*	*No*	*Yes*	*No*
Positioning map and table	*Locating point*	*Yes*	*Yes*	*Yes*	*Yes*
Point-symbol maps	*Locating point*	*Yes*	*Yes*	*Yes*	*Yes*
Point density maps	*Statistical region and locating point*	*Yes*	*No*	*Yes*	*No*

Fig. 1. Relationships between statistical attributes and its representing approaches for thematic maps

For the latter (ii), a typical mapping approach for further analysis is interpolation, including famous IDW (Inverse Distance Weight) interpolation, Empirical Bayesian Kriging interpolation, Moving Window Kriging interpolation, etc. Taking the famous IDW interpolation for example, it explicitly implements that things those are close to one another are more alike than those that are farther apart. To predict a value for any unmeasured location, IDW uses the measured values surrounding the prediction location. The measured values close to the prediction location have more influence on the predicted value than those farther away, so IDW gives greater weights to points closer to the prediction location, and the weights diminish as a function of distance, hence the name Inverse Distance Weighted.

It also should be noticed that, the scales of data are closed associated with both (i) final thematic cartographic visualization for former analysis (where data scales are abstracted from statistic attributes/indicators) and (ii) approach for further analysis (typically only numerical data rather than categorical data is allowed for interpolation). Overall, the scales of data could be categorized into four types, i.e., nominal-scale, sequence-scale, interval-scale, ratio-scale. In detail, it is regarded that: (1) the main characteristics of nominal-scale data is describing the difference between classes or distinguishes in quality, e.g., in daily life, people are distinguished by different names, and names are nominal-scale data; (2) and the main characteristics of sequence-scale data is data not only able to be differentiated but also able to be ordered by a certain sequence, e.g., everyone grow from young, to middle-aged, finally to old; (3) furthermore, interval-scale data is data which could be both sequenced by order and calculated by operator '−', in another word, the interval between adjacent levels (also called grades, hierarchies) could be described using operator '−', e.g., the temperature of place A is 15° and that of place B is 5°, then it can be inferred that A has a 10-degree higher temperature than B, while the statement that A has a temperature as triple as B is meaningless; (4) based on the above, ratio-scale data is data able to be calculated using operator '−', '+' and '/' which has the absolute 'zero' point, e.g., the population of place A is 10,000 and that of place B is 5,000, then it can be inferred that A has a population twice as B.

The conversion direction from high-level data scale to low-level data scale is unidirectional, which is shown in Fig. 2. In another word, the high-level scale data could be easily converted into low-level scale because the former could be regarded as an implicit latter (i.e., sequence-scale data is an implicit instance of nominal-scale data, interval-scale data is an implicit instance of sequence-scale data, and ratio-scale data is an implicit instance of interval-scale data); by contrast, the latter could only be transformed into the former with additional information.

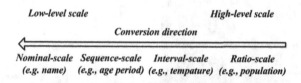

Fig. 2. The conversion direction between different scale data

It should also be noticed that, the data scale mentioned here is also closely associated with pre-analysis process for spatial cluster analysis, because in most cases of spatial cluster analysis only ratio-scale data are allowed while nominal-scale data is only permitted in several data cluster approaches.

It is regarded here that, for nominal- or sequencing-scale, disparate colors are helpful in identifying quality discrepancies between point-based features intuitively, and for interval- or ratio-scale data, color gradients or brightness levels can be used to portray their hierarchies or levels.

4 Case Study

Here, empirical data is employed for case study especially for disease mapping following related laws in China. More specifically, "Law of the People's Republic of China on Prevention and Treatment of Infectious Diseases" (abbreviated as "PTID Law" later) was enacted and published in 1989, in order to prevent, control and put an end to the outbreak and spread of infectious diseases and to ensure the health of the people and public sanitation in China [11]. In "PTID Law", it says that, the infectious diseases governed by this law are divided into Classes A, B and C order by harm degree. In detail, it exist 2 types of infectious diseases under Class A including plague and cholera, 25 types of infectious diseases under Class B including infectious SARS, AIDS, viral hepatitis, etc., and 10 types of infectious diseases C including influenza, epidemic parotitis, etc.

Based on this law, empirical data from in Ningbo City, Zhejiang Province, China is employed. Ningbo city is a city specifically designated in the state plan which has a 7.825 million population (up to 2015) and a 9,816 square kilometers area located at the east of China. More specifically, three-level administrative delimitation of Ningbo city is shown in Fig. 3, i.e., in level 1 shown in Fig. 3(a) the spatial location of Ningbo city in China is given, in level 2 shown in Fig. 3(b) boundaries of 11 districts/counties/county-level cities in Ningbo are given, and in level 3 shown in Fig. 3(c) boundaries of 153 streets/towns/villages in each district/county/county-level city are delimited where 'C' is short for 'county-level City', 'D' is short for 'District' and 'Co' is short for 'County' in level 2, 'S' is short for 'Street', 'T' is short for 'Town' and 'V' is short for 'Village' in level 3.

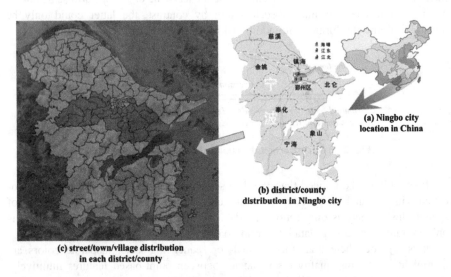

(a) Ningbo city location in China

(b) district/county distribution in Ningbo city

(c) street/town/village distribution in each district/county

Fig. 3. Three-level administrative delimitation for Ningbo City

These epidemiological data belongs to 2011-year Ningbo epidemiological data which has been collected up to now whose statistic attributes come from relevant departments (e.g., hospitals, disease control center) where involved epidemiology types in Ningbo are ticked in Fig. 4. Correspondingly, spatial locations for collected records are extracted from the 'address' field referencing the widely-used geo-portal TianDiTu (http://www.nbmap.gov.cn) where the whole process is often abbreviated as 'geocoding'. It should be noticed that, due to the lack of partial fields (especially the

Infectious Diseases under Class A	Infectious Diseases Under Class B		Infectious Diseases Under Class C
plague	*pertussis* ✓	*typhoid and*	*influenza* ✓
cholera	*measles* ✓	*paratyphoid* ✓	*epidemic parotitis* ✓
	viral heptitis ✓	*epidemic*	*rubella*
	gonorrhoea ✓	*hemorrhagic fever*	*leprosy*
	malaria ✓	*bacillary and*	*Kala-azar*
	syphilis ✓	*amebic dysentery*	*filariasis*
	diphtheria	*pulmonary*	*echinococcosis*
	tetanus infantum	*tuberculosis*	*epidemic and*
	scarlet fever	*highly pathogenic*	*endemic typhus*
	rabies	*avian influenza*	*acuate hemorrhagic*
Note: epidemic	*poliomyelitis*	*epidemic*	*conjunctivitis* ✓
types involved	*brucellosis*	*cerebrospinal*	*Infectious diarrhea*
in case study in	*dengue fever*	*meningitis*	*other than cholera,*
Ningbo are	*anthrax*	*epidemic*	*bacillary and amebic*
labeled as ticks	*leptospirosis*	*encephalitis B*	*dysentery, typhoid*
here	*schistosomiasis*		*and paratyphoid* ✓
	infectious SARS		
	AIDS		

Fig. 4. Disease types involved in Ningbo City from 2011 to 2013

'address' field), up to now only 1891 records from original thousands of records could be successfully geocoded.

Using the above epidemiology data with its spatial location and the proposed cartography approach taking data scale into account, commercial GIS software ESRI ArcGIS is employed for final visualization implementation. And the chosen fields for cartography are listed as follows: the occurring district, the age, the gender, the career, the disease category, the disease type.

(1) the 1st attribute (i.e., the occurring district, belonging to nominal-scale data) covers 9 items under administration of Ningbo: JiangBei district, JiangDong district, HaiShu district, Yinzhou district, BeiLun district, FengHua city, XiangShan county, YuYao city, CityXi city, Ninghai county and ZhenHai district; (2) the 2nd attribute (i.e., the age, belonging to ratio-scale data) ranges from 1 to 100, here gives a typical group for age 1–100: 1–10 year old, 11–20 year old, 21–30 year old, 31–40 year old, 41–50 year old, 51–60 year old, 61–70 year old, 71–80 year old, 81–90 year old and 91–100 year old; (3) the 3rd attribute (i.e., the gender, belonging to nominal-scale data) covers 2 items: the male and the female; (4) the 4th attribute (i.e., the career, belonging to nominal-scale data) covers 14 items which are closely associated with the infectious diseases: the residentially- scattered children, the childcare children, the students (in primary, junior and senior scales), restaurant and food service people, the commercial service people, the hospital staffs, the cadre staffs, the workers, the farmer, the rural laborer, the teacher, the retired people, unemployed people and others; (5) the 5th attribute (i.e., the disease category, belonging to sequence-scale data) covers 3 sequences order by harm degree in accordance with PTID Law as mentioned above: the infectious diseases under Class A (owning the high-level harm), the infectious diseases under Class B (owning the medium-level harm), the infectious diseases under Class C (owning the low-level harm); (6) the 6th attribute (i.e., the disease type, belonging to

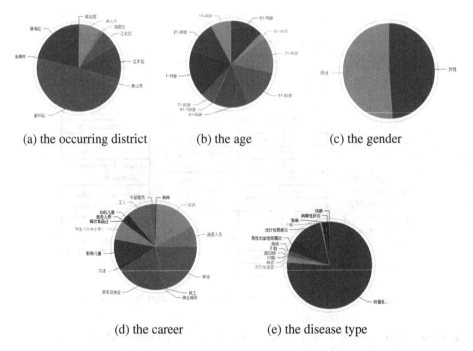

(a) the occurring district   (b) the age   (c) the gender

(d) the career   (e) the disease type

Fig. 5. Traditional statistics for attributes of epidemic data

nominal-scale data) covers 11 types which could be easily found in Ningbo city: viral hepatitis, measles, typhoid and paratyphoid, pertussis, gonorrhea, syphilis, malaria, influenza, epidemic parotitis, acute hemorrhagic conjunctivitis, infectious diarrhea other than cholera, bacillary and amebic dysentery, typhoid and paratyphoid;

The statistics for the above attributes using traditional approaches (e.g., pie diagrams) are shown in Fig. 5(a)–(e) which provides percentage of components for each attribute where corresponding spatial distribution is lacked.

By contrast, disease cartography for above attributes using categorized or quantitized thematic mapping taking efficient cartography for different data scales into account is given in Fig. 6(a)–(f).

(1) in Fig. 6(a), taking cartography for 'occurring district' owning nominal-scale into account, categorized thematic mapping is employed, and it could be easily found from the map that, the most epidemiology cases occur in Yinzhou district, Jiangdong district and Zhenhai district (ticked at the left legend) which could not be observed using traditional statistic approach in Fig. 5(a);

(2) in Fig. 6(b), taking cartography for 'age' owning ratio-scale into account, quantitized thematic mapping is employed, and it could be easily found from the map that, in the urban area of Ningbo city including Haishu district, Jiangbei district, Jiangdong district, Yinzhou district the age is distributed in a relatively homogeneous pattern while that in Xiangshan county is gathering at the young period which could not be observed using traditional statistic approach in Fig. 5(b);

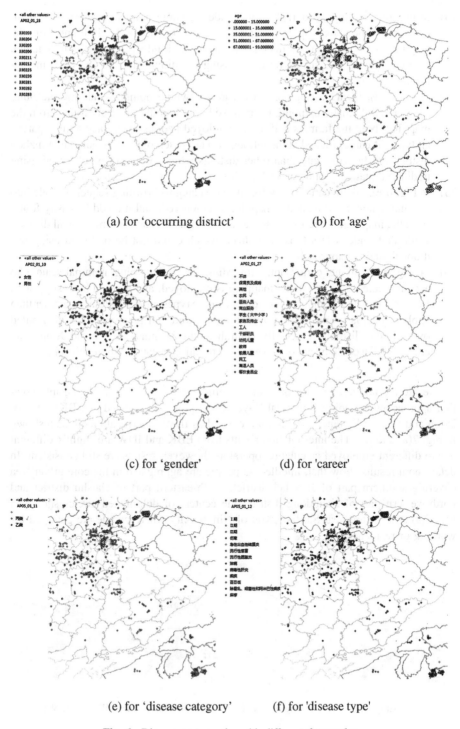

(a) for 'occurring district'   (b) for 'age'

(c) for 'gender'   (d) for 'career'

(e) for 'disease category'   (f) for 'disease type'

Fig. 6. Disease cartography with different data scales

(3) in Fig. 6(c), taking cartography for 'gender' owning nominal-scale into account, categorized thematic mapping is employed, and it could be easily found from the map that, more male than female are prone to catch infectious disease in Yinzhou district which could not be observed using traditional statistic approach in Figure in Fig. 5(c);

(4) in Fig. 6(d), taking cartography for 'career' owning nominal-scale into account, categorized thematic mapping is employed, and it could be easily found from the map that, both the farmers and the unemployed people which take a huge part in all types of career (ticked at the left legend) are much more distributed in Yinzhou district and Fenghua city than other districts which could not be observed using traditional statistic approach in Fig. 5(d);

(5) in Fig. 6(e), taking cartography for 'disease category' owning sequence-scale into account, categorized thematic mapping is employed, and it could be easily found from the map that, infectious diseases under Class B is decentralized in all districts while that under Class C is centralized which could not be observed using traditional statistic approach;

(6) in Fig. 6(f), taking cartography for 'disease type' owning nominal-scale into account, categorized thematic mapping is employed, and it could be easily found from the map that, compared with other disease types, infectious diarrhea other than cholera, bacillary and amebic dysentery, typhoid and paratyphoid is distributed over all the districts, especially centralized in Zhenhai district and Xiangshan county which could be not observed using traditional statistic approach in Fig. 5(e);

Beside the above thematic mapping for different data scales, employed interpolation approaches including Empirical Bayesian Kriging (abbreviated as EBK) interpolation and Inverse Distance Weight (abbreviated as IDW) interpolation are also shown in Fig. 7(a) and (b). The interpolation results from EBK and IDW are slightly different due to different employed calculation operators, however, results are still consistent. In detail, both results show that, middle-age people are aggregated in the core urban area covering southern part of Jiangbei district, north-eastern part of Haishu district and north-western part of Jiangdong district (the centers of delimitated circles shown in Fig. 7(a) and (b) are near SanJiangKou of Ningbo city where people are gathered for working or residence).

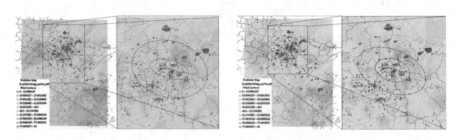

(a) Empirical Bayesian Kriging (EBK)   (b) Inverse Distance Weight (IDW)

Fig. 7. Interpolation of epidemiology data

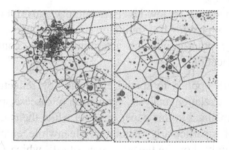

Fig. 8. Voronoi for hospitals and health-care sites in Ningbo City

In addition to thematic cartography and interpolation, more functions could be provided by GIS for spatial epidemiology study, e.g., using Voronoi diagrams to judge whether the location of hospital and health-care sites are distributed reasonably as shown in Fig. 8, e.g., if more people who have caught infectious diseases in the region delimitated by Voronoi prefer to going to obtain health care or treatment in the surrounding regions, it could be tentatively make a judgment that the hospital/health-care site in this region is not set reasonably in the space domain which should be paid more attention to later by decision makers.

5 Conclusion

Using the technologies shown above, clinical significances also have been found as follows:

(i)   low-aged children and students appear in the top distribution of measles, bacillary and amebic dysentery, influenza, epidemic parotitis, acute hemorrhagic conjunctivitis, other infectious diarrhea, where efforts on prevention and treatment on related places (typically in kindergartens, primary schools) should be paid more attention to. Furthermore, strong correlation between the above types of infectious diseases and kindergartens and schools will be verified from the spatial perspective where spatial technologies such as spatial buffering, point-in-polygon determination, etc. could be employed;

(ii) for gonorrhea and syphilis, although distribution ranking of both age and profession are different, their distribution sets of age and profession are the same, so it could be easily guessed that it also exists strong correlation for spatial distribution between gonorrhea and syphilis where spatial technologies such as spatial buffering, spatial overlapping, etc. could be employed for further verification;

(iii) patients of other infectious diarrhea takes up the most (nearly 70 %) in those of all types of infectious diseases, and the age distribution for other infectious diarrhea mainly ranges from 41 to 65 year old which shows a great significance that middle-aged group is much more prone to catch other infectious diarrhea than young citizens and old citizens, and it could also be guessed that this maybe contribute from eating in low-level restaurants and night snacks in sidewalk snack vendors both having bad sanitation conditions where spatial analysis using spatial buffering, point-in-polygon determination, etc. could also be employed for further verification;

So, the role of GIS applied to spatial epidemiology reflecting in spatial cluster analysis, spatial auto-correlation analysis, simulation of disease spreading process, and disease mapping is explained in this paper in detail while thematic cartography taking data scale into account is particularly elaborated. Meanwhile, empirical data of Ningbo City is used for case study showing the advantage of GIS which could not be observed using traditional statistic approaches. In further work, spatial cluster analysis, especially grid-based spatial cluster following the principle of "data compression", beneficial to intuitively find hot regions or cold regions of patient individuals, will be devoted to

Acknowledgments. This work is supported by Open Research Fund of State Key Laboratory of Information Engineering in Surveying, Mapping and Remote Sensing (15I03) and Natural Science Foundation in China (No. 41601428, 41301439). The authors would like to thank both Health and Family Planning Commission of Ningbo Municipality and Ningbo Zhongjing Technology Development Limited Cooperation for providing the experimental epidemic data.

References

1. Andritsos, P.: Data clustering techniques. Digital Image Process. 1–34 (2002)
2. Anselin, L.: Local indicators of spatial association_LISA. Geogr. Anal. **27**(2), 93–115 (1995)
3. Bouguettaya, A., Viet, Q.L.: Data clustering analysis in a multi-dimensional space. Inf. Sci. **112**(s1–4), 267–295 (1998)
4. Elliiot, P., Wakefield, J.C., Best, N.G., Briggs, D.J.: Spatial Epidemiology: Methods and Applications. Oxford University Press, USA (2000)
5. Guo, R.Z.: Spatial characteristics of interval-scaled and ratio-scaled geo-data and their influence on graphic representation. Map **3**, 3–7 (1987). (in Chinese)
6. Guo, R.Z.: Spatial Analysis. High Education Press, Beijing (2001). (in Chinese)
7. Hu, T., Du, Q.Y., Ren, F., Liang, S., Lin, D.N., Li, J.J., Chen, Y.: Spatial analysis of the home addresses of hospital patients with hepatitis B infection or hepatoma in Shenzhen, China from 2010 to 2012. Int. J. Environ. Res. Public Health **11**(3), 3143–3155 (2014)
8. Hu, Y., Bergquist, R., Lynn, H., Gao, F.H., et al.: Sandwich mapping of schistosomiasis risk in Anhui Province, China. Geospatial Health **10**, 324 (2015)
9. Jain, A.K., Law, M.H.: Data clustering: a user's dilemma. In: Pal, S.K., Bandyopadhyay, S., Biswas, S. (eds.) PReMI 2005. LNCS, vol. 3776, pp. 1–10. Springer, Heidelberg (2005). doi:10.1007/11590316_1
10. Koua, E.L., Krark, M.J.: Geovisualization to support the exploration of large health and demographic survey data. Int. J. Health Geogr. **3**, 12 (2004)
11. Law of the People's Republic of China on Prevention and Treatment of Infectious Diseases. Order No. 5 of the President of the People's Republic of China (2013)
12. Li, J., Alem, L., Huang, W.: Supporting frontline health workers through the use of a mobile collaboration tool. In: Yin, X., Ho, K., Zeng, D., Aickelin, U., Zhou, R., Wang, H. (eds.) HIS 2015. LNCS, vol. 9085, pp. 31–36. Springer, Heidelberg (2015). doi:10.1007/978-3-319-19156-0_4

13. Li, L., Xi, Y.L., Ren, F.: Spatio-temporal distribution characteristics and trajectory similarity analysis of tuberculosis in Beijing, China. Int. J. Environ. Res. Public Health **13**(291), 17 p. (2016)
14. Liu, H.K., Tang, M.: A review on global epidemics spreading. Complex Syst. Complex. Sci. **8**(3), 86–94 (2011). (in Chinese)
15. Liu, Q.L., Li, Z.L., Deng, M., Tang, J.B., Mei, X.M.: Modeling the effect of scale on clustering of spatial points. Comput. Environ. Urban Syst. **52**, 81–92 (2015)
16. Rodriguez-Morales, A.J., Orrego-Acevedo, C.A., Zambrano-Munoz, Y., et al.: Mapping malaria in municipalities of the coffee triangle region of Columbia using geographic information systems. J. Infect. Public Health **8**, 603–611 (2015)
17. Wang, Y.X., Du, Q.Y., Ren, F., Liang, S., Lin, D.N., Tian, Q., Chen, Y., Li, J.J.: Spatio-temporal variation and prediction of ischemic heart disease hospitalization in Shenzhen, China. Int. J. Environ. Res. Public Health **11**(5), 4799–4824 (2014)
18. Wang, Z.S.: Research of disease mapping over small-area based on spatial model. Ph.D. Dissertation, Wuhan University, Wuhan (2014). (in Chinese)
19. Wang, Z.S., Du, Q.Y., Liang, S., Nie, K., Lin, D.N., Chen, Y., Li, J.J.: Analysis of the spatial variation of hospitalization admissions for hypertension disease in Shenzhen, China. Int. J. Environ. Res. Public Health **11**(1), 713–733 (2014)
20. Ward, H., Iverson, J., Law, M., Maher, L.: Quilt plots: a simple tool for the visualization of large epidemiological data. PLoS ONE **9**(1), e85047 (2014)
21. Xi, Y.L., Ren, F., Liang, S., Zhang, J.H., Lin, D.N.: Spatial analysis of the distribution, risk factors and access to medical resources and patients with hepatitis B in Shenzhen, China. Int. J. Environ. Res. Public Health **11**(11), 11505–11527 (2014)
22. Xiang, F., Guan, W., Huang, X., Fan, X., Cai, Y., Yu, H.: Mobile clinical scale collection system for in-hospital stroke patient assessments using Html5 technology. In: Yin, X., Ho, K., Zeng, D., Aickelin, U., Zhou, R., Wang, H. (eds.) HIS 2015. LNCS, vol. 9085, pp. 185–194. Springer, Heidelberg (2015). doi:10.1007/978-3-319-19156-0_19
23. Yu, C.B., Ren, F., Du, Q.Y., Zhao, Z.Y., Nie, K.: Web map-based POI visualization for spatial decision support. Cartography Geogr. Inf. Sci. **40**(3), 172–181 (2013)
24. Yu, L., Xue, H.F., Li, G.: Research of epidemic spread model. Comput. Simul. **24**(4), 57–60 (2007). (in Chinese)
25. Zaïane, O.R., Foss, A., Lee, C.-H., Wang, W.: On data clustering analysis: scalability, constraints, and validation. In: Chen, M.-S., Yu, P.S., Liu, B. (eds.) PAKDD 2002. LNCS (LNAI), vol. 2336, pp. 28–39. Springer, Heidelberg (2002). doi:10.1007/3-540-47887-6_4
26. Zeng, X.G., Du, Q.Y., et al.: Design and implementation of a web interactive thematic cartography method based on a web service chain. Bol. Cienc. Geod. **19**(2), 172–190 (2013). sec. Artigos, Curitiba
27. Zhang, K.Q., Guo, R.Z.: Mathematical Models for Thematic Cartography. Survey and Mapping Press, Beijing (1988). (in Chinese)
28. Zhao, F.: Research on smart visualization and online interactive mapping model of thematic cartography. Ph.D. Dissertation, Wuhan University, Wuhan (2012). (in Chinese)
29. Zhou, X.N.: Spatial Epidemiology[M]. Science Press, Beijing (2009). (in Chinese)

Differential Feature Recognition of Breast Cancer Patients Based on Minimum Spanning Tree Clustering and F-statistics

Juanying Xie[✉], Ying Li, Ying Zhou, and Mingzhao Wang

School of Computer Science, Shaanxi Normal University,
Xi'an 710062, People's Republic of China
xiejuany@snnu.edu.cn

Abstract. The differential feature recognition algorithm of breast cancer patients is presented in this paper based on minimum spanning tree (MST) and F-statistics. The algorithm uses the minimum spanning tree clustering algorithm to cluster features of breast cancer data and the F-statistics to determine the proper number of feature clusters. Features most relevant to class labels are selected from each feature cluster to comprise the differential features. After that, samples with recognized features are clustered via MST clustering algorithm. The validity of our algorithm is evaluated by its clustering accuracy on breast cancer dataset of WDBC. In the experiments, correlations between features and class labels and similarities between features are measured by the cosine similarity and Pearson correlation coefficient. Similarities between samples are measured by the cosine similarity, the Euclidean distance and the Pearson correlation coefficient. Experimental results show that the highest clustering accuracy can be got when the cosine similarity is used to measure correlations between features and class labels and similarities between features while the Euclidean distance is used to measure similarities between samples. The recognized features are: mean radius, mean fractal dimension and standard error of fractal dimension.

Keywords: F-statistic · Minimum spanning tree (MST) · Clustering · Breast cancer · Feature recognition

1 Introduction

Breast cancer is one of malignant tumors which develops from breast tissue. The morbidity has been increasing rapidly in China in the past decades. It is reported that the 10 years survival rates of breast cancer patients in stages T4, T3, T2, T1 are 19.7 %, 46.0 %, 62.6 % and 87.8 % respectively [1]. The situation of breast cancer is very serious, though the pathogenic factors are still vague. Feature recognition can be used for selecting representative features. The recognition rate of breast cancer patients can be improved by using the representative features other than using the original features. The selected representative features can also be used by medicine doctors to make the clinical diagnosis and decions. An efficient fast clustering-based feature subset selection algorithm [2] clustered features using minimum spanning tree

© Springer International Publishing AG 2016
X. Yin et al. (Eds.): HIS 2016, LNCS 10038, pp. 194–204, 2016.
DOI: 10.1007/978-3-319-48335-1_21

clustering algorithm, and selected features from each cluster, so that the features which are strongly related to the class label can be found to form a feature subset. However, the Symmetric Uncertainty (SU) used in the algorithm [2] cannot measure the similarity between variables with unknown entropies. In this study, we propose a differential feature recognition algorithm based on minimum spanning tree and F-statistics. Our algorithm will group features into clusters based on minimum spanning tree clustering algorithm, and the representative features are selected from each cluster according to the strong correlation between them and the class labels. The similarities between variables is measured via cosine similarity and Pearson correlation coefficient. The optimal number of feature clusters is determined by F-statistics.

2   Related Algorithms and Concepts

2.1   The Minimum Spanning Tree Clustering Algorithm

The minimum spanning tree clustering algorithm (MST) [3] can find the acyclic sub-graph with the minimum weight from a connected weighted graph with n nodes. There are two types of MST algorithm. The first one is Prim algorithm, and the other one is Kruskal algorithm. Prim algorithm performs better on the dense graph while Kruskal algorithm does better on the sparse graph. In this paper, the breast cancer data WDBC is large, hence we choose the Prim algorithm to cluster features of breast cancer. We construct the MST of features by using features as nodes of a graph and the similarities between features as weights between related nodes.

2.2   F-statistics

F-statistics [4–7] obeys F distribution whose curve goes up first, then falls. F-statistics can be used to evaluate whether the clustering is good enough or not. The clustering is good when the objects in the same cluster are related to each other and those in different clusters are relatively independent. The higher the F-statistics is, the better the clustering is. The number of clusters will be optimized when the F-statistics of the clustering reaches its highest value. The F-statistics is defined in Eq. (1).

$$F = \frac{\sum_{j=1}^{k} n_j \left\| \bar{x}^{(j)} - \bar{x} \right\|^2 \Big/ (k-1)}{\sum_{j=1}^{k} \sum_{i=1}^{n_j} \left\| x_i^{(j)} - \bar{x}^{(j)} \right\|^2 \Big/ (n-k)} \tag{1}$$

Where, k is the number of clusters. j is the jth cluster. $\bar{x}^{(j)}$ is the centroid of the jth cluster. $\bar{x}$ is the centroid of all data set. n is the number of objects in the data set, n_j is the number of objects in the jth cluster. $\left\| \bar{x}^{(j)} - \bar{x} \right\|$ is the distance between the centroid of the jth cluster and the centroid of all data set. $\left\| x_i^{(j)} - \bar{x}^{(j)} \right\|$ is the distance between the object i of the jth cluster and the centroid of jth cluster.

2.3 Similarity Metrics

The similarity is to measure how close between two objects. In this study, we use the cosine similarity and Pearson correlation coefficient to measure the similarities between features, and also use them to measure the similarities between features and class labels. We use cosine similarity, Pearson correlation coefficient and Euclidean distance to measure the similarity between samples. For two n dimensional variables $\mathbf{X}(x_1, x_2, x_3 \ldots x_n)$ and $\mathbf{Y}(y_1, y_2, y_3 \ldots y_n)$, the definition of Euclidean distance, cosine similarity and Pearson correlation coefficient are defined in (2)–(4) [8].

$$d(\mathbf{X}, \mathbf{Y}) = \sqrt{\sum_{k=1}^{n} (x_k - y_k)^2} \tag{2}$$

$$\cos(\mathbf{X}, \mathbf{Y}) = \frac{\mathbf{X} \cdot \mathbf{Y}}{\|\mathbf{X}\| \cdot \|\mathbf{Y}\|} \tag{3}$$

$$corr(\mathbf{X}, \mathbf{Y}) = \frac{\sum\limits_{k=1}^{n} (x_k - \bar{x})(y_k - \bar{y})}{\sqrt{\sum\limits_{k=1}^{n} (x_k - \bar{x})^2 \sum\limits_{k=1}^{n} (y_k - \bar{y})^2}} \tag{4}$$

Where, $\bar{x}$ is the mean value of $\mathbf{X}$, and $\bar{y}$ is the mean value of $\mathbf{Y}$.

3 Our Feature Recognition Algorithm Based on MST Clustering Algorithm and F-statistics

We first cluster features of breast cancers by using MST clustering algorithm, then select features which are strongly related to the class labels from each cluster to form the recognition feature subset. The cosine similarity and Pearson correlation coefficient are adopted to measure the similarities between variables in our feature recognition algorithm. In order to get k feature clusters, we need to cut the $k-1$ edges with last $k-1$ similarities. In order to determine the optimum number k of feature clusters, we use F-statistics to find it, that is to value how many feature clusters will be the optimal number of feature clusters. The details of our algorithm are shown as follows.

3.1 Data Pre-processing

We measure the similarities between features by Pearson correlation coefficient and cosine similarity to get the similarity matrix of features. The original number of features is n.

3.2 Cluster the Features of Breast Cancer Data by MST Clustering Algorithm

- We construct the graph with features as nodes and the similarity values between features as weight of edges between related nodes. MST is constructed by using Prim algorithm for the graph of features.
- In order to get the $k(k = 2, 3, \ldots, m - 1, m, m + 1, \ldots, n)$ clusters of features, the $k-1$ edges with last $k-1$ weights are to be cut.

3.3 Determine the Optimized Number of Clusters via F-Statistics

- Calculate the F-statistics F_k $(k = 2, 3, \ldots, m - 1, m, m + 1, \ldots, n)$ for the clustering with k feature clusters.
- Estimate whether the value of F_k reaches the largest value F_m or not, that is $F_{m-1} < F_m > F_{m+1} > F_{m+2}$. If the value of F_k has not reached the highest value F_m, then add 1 to k, and go to the second step of Subsect. 3.2 until F_k reach the highest value F_m. If F_k reaches the highest value F_m, then m is the optimized number of feature clusters.

3.4 Recognize Features from Each Cluster

- Measure the correlation between features and class labels via cosine similarity measurement and Pearson correlation coefficient after the optimum number of feature clusters m has been found.
- Select one representative feature from each cluster, so that the selected features are strongly related to class labels.
- All of the representative features constitute the differential feature subset for tell breast cancer patients from normal people.

4 Data Set and Experimental Design

4.1 Breast Cancer Data Set

The breast cancer data set WDBC [9] used in our experiment is taken from the UCI machine learning repository. It includes 569 samples, 32 attributes (ID, diagnosis, and 30 real-valued input features), that is $U = \{x_1, x_2, x_3, \cdots, x_{569}\}$, $x_i = \{x_{i_{ID}}, x_{i_{Diagnosis}}, x_{i_1}, x_{i_2}, x_{i_3}, \cdots, x_{i_{30}}\}$. This data set doesn't miss any attribute values. The information of 30 real-valued features is shown in Table 1.

Table 1. Breast cancer Wisconsin (Diagnostic) data set

Breast Cancer (number of patients)	Features	
Benign (357)	Feature 1: Means of radius	Feature 16: Standard error of compactness
Malignant (212)	Feature 2: Means of texture	Feature 17: Standard error of concavity
	Feature 3: Means of perimeter	Feature 18: Standard error of concave points
	Feature 4: Means of area	Feature 19: Standard error of symmetry
	Feature 5: Means of smoothness	Feature 20: Standard error of fractal dimension
	Feature 6: Means of compactness	Feature 21: Mean of the three largest values of radius
	Feature 7: Means of concavity	Feature 22: Mean of the three largest values of texture
	Feature 8: Means of concave points	Feature 23: Mean of the three largest values of perimeter
	Feature 9: Means of symmetry	Feature 24: Mean of the three largest values of area
	Feature 10: Means of fractal dimension	Feature 25: Mean of the three largest values of smoothness
	Feature 11: Standard error of radius	Feature 26: Mean of the three largest values of compactness
	Feature 12: Standard error of texture	Feature 27: Mean of the three largest values of concavity
	Feature 13: Standard error of perimeter	Feature 28: Mean of the three largest values of concave points
	Feature 14: Standard error of area	Feature 29: Mean of the three largest values of symmetry
	Feature 15: Standard error of smoothness	Feature 30: Mean of the three largest values of fractal dimension

4.2   Experimental Procedures

We load the breast cancer data set first, then use our feature recognition algorithm to recognize those representative features. Where we first construct the graph with features as nodes and with the similarities between features as weight of edges between nodes, then we use Prim algorithm to find the MST of the feature graph, during which the optimum number of feature clusters are determined via F-statistics. After the optimal clustering is found, we choose the representative features from each feature cluster, so that the selected features are strongly related to class labels. In order to evaluate our algorithm, we compare the clustering accuracy of our algorithm on the breast cancer data set where each sample has the representative features with those where the breast cancer samples with all of the original features. Sample similarities are calculated via the cosine similarity, Euclidean distance and Pearson correlation coefficient respectively when finding the clustering of samples. We do the sample clustering via the Prim algorithm, and the edge with the minimum value is cut off to get two sample clusters. After we get two sample clusters, calculate the clustering accuracy. The procedure of our experiment is shown in Fig. 1.

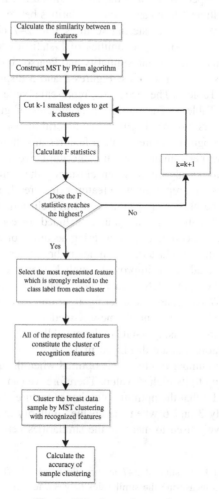

Fig. 1. Experimental procedure

5   Experimental Results and the Analysis

This experiment uses cosine similarity and Pearson correlation coefficient to measure the similarities between features. We group features of breast cancer via MST clustering algorithm while using F-statistics to find the optimum number of feature clusters. When we get the optimal clusters of features, the representative features are selected from each cluster to construct the selected feature subset. We respectively use the cosine similarity and Pearson similarity metrics to measure the correlation between features and class labels when we are to select the representative features from each feature cluster. After the representative features are found, we group samples only with the representative features for each sample in the breast cancer data set into two clusters via MST clustering algorithm while respectively using the cosine similarity, Euclidean distance and Pearson correlation coefficient to measure the similarities between samples.

The experimental results of clustering features into 2–7 clusters are shown in Table 2, including the corresponding quantities of F-statistics for the related feature clustering respectively using the cosine similarity and Pearson correlation coefficient to measure the similarities between features. Figures 2 and 3 display the corresponding curves of F-statistics in Table 2. The recognized representative features of breast cancer data set are shown in Table 3. The clustering accuracies of grouping breast cancer samples into two clusters via MST clustering algorithm using different similarity metrics and different recognized representative features are shown in Table 4.

In order to test the performance of our algorithm, we compare the clustering accuracy of MST clustering algorithm when clustering the samples of breast cancer data set into two clusters with representative features (features 1, 10 and 20) recognized by our algorithm and the clustering accuracy of MST clustering algorithm on breast cancer data set with all of the original features included for each sample, denoted as MST_All. Furthermore, we compare the clustering accuracy of our study with that of other clustering algorithms on clustering samples in breast cancer data set with all of the original features, including an improved rough K-means clustering algorithm in [10] shorted as RK, and weighted KNN Data Classification Algorithm Based on Rough Set in [11] denoted as W-KNN, and a clustering algorithm based on local center object in [12] simply expressed as LCO, and the new K-medoids clustering algorithm based on granular computing in [13] using K-GC to denote. All of clustering accuracies of the compared clustering algorithms are displayed in Table 5.

It is known that the number of clusters is optimal when the quantity of F-statistics of that clustering goes up to its highest value. Therefore we can see from the results in Table 2 and Figs. 2 and 3 that the optimum number of feature clusters of breast cancer data set are respectively 3 and 6 when the cosine similarity and Pearson correlation coefficient are respectively used to measure the similarities between features.

Table 2. The quantity of F-statistics of 2–7 feature clusters by MST clustering algorithm in different similarity metrics measuring the similarities between features

The number of clusters	F-statistics	
	Cosine similarity	Pearson correlation coefficient
2	0.0917	0.0881
3	**0.3639**	0.0612
4	0.2687	0.1845
5	0.2182	0.7235
6	0.1868	**0.9113**
7	0.1646	0.7496

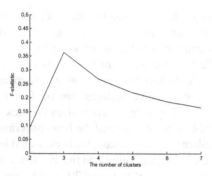

Fig. 2. The curve of F-statistics for clustering features into 2–7 clusters by MST using cosine similarity metric to measure the similarities between features

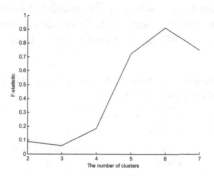

Fig. 3. The curve of F-statistic for clustering features into 2–7 clusters by MST using Pearson correlated coefficient to measure the similarities between features

Table 3. The representative features of breast cancer via different similarity metrics

	The optimal number of clusters	The No. of representative features	
		The correlation between features and class labels measured by cosine similarity	The correlation between features and class labels measured by Pearson correlation coefficient
The similarity between features measured by cosine similarity	3	1; 10; 20	20; 23; 28
The similarity between features measured by Pearson correlation coefficient	6	3; 9; 10; 21; 23; 30	1; 3; 13; 21; 23; 28

From the results in Table 3, we can see that the selected representative features are not always same when the different similarity metrics are used to measure the similarities between features and the correlations between features and class labels. It can also be seen from the Table 3 that there are three features can be found as representative features when the similarities between features are measured via cosine similarity, and there are 6 representative features can be found when the similarities between features are measured by Pearson correlation coefficient.

From the results in Table 4, we can see that the best clustering accuracy has been got is 79.96 % when the similarities between samples is measured in Euclidean distance to group samples via MST clustering algorithm into two clusters while each sample is only with selected representative features of 1,10, and 20. These three representative features are found by both using the cosine similarity measurement to measure the similarities between features and the correlations between features and class labels when doing feature selection via MST and F-statistics. Therefore we can say that features 1, 10, and 20 consititute the optimal feature subset to distinguish the breast cancer patients from normal people. The information of features 1, 10 and 20 are mean radius, mean fractal dimension and standard error of fractal dimension, respectively.

Table 4. The clustering accuracies of breast cancer samples by MST clustering algorithm using the original features and the representative features

The no. of representative features (similarity metrics between features and between features and class labels when finding the representative features)	Clustering accuracy		
	Similarity between samples measured by cosine similarity	Similarity between samples measured by Euclidean distance	Similarity between samples measured by Pearson correlation coefficient
Original 30 features	0.7399	0.6573	0.6960
1, 10, 20 (both by cosine similarity)	0.6274	**0.7996**	0.6274
20; 23; 28 (respectively by cosine similarity and Pearson correlation coefficient)	0.7241	0.7557	0.7381
1, 3, 13, 21, 23, 28 (both by Pearson correlation coefficient)	0.7452	0.7698	0.7399
3; 9; 10; 21; 23; 30 (respectively by Pearson correlation coefficient and cosine similarity)	0.7170	0.7733	0.7206

Table 5. Accuracy of WDBC clustering with different algorithms

Algorithm	RK	W-KNN	LCO	K-GC	This study	MST_All
The number of features	30	30	30	30	3	30
Accuracy	94.475 %	96.25 %	77.2 %	85.41 %	79.96 %	65.73 %

The results in Table 5 show that the clustering accuracy of MST algorithm is improved more than 14 % using the only three representative features found by our algorithm than using the all of 30 original features. Although the clustering accuracy of our work is not the highest one, it is still a comparative one compared to those of available algorithms with all of the original features without any feature selection process because our study only uses the 10 % features of the original ones.

Therefore, our study can reduce the dimensions of breast cancer data set to its 10 %, which not only reduce the necessary storage for data set, but also help the medicine doctors to make the clinic decision with only three features of mean radius, mean fractal dimension and standard error of fractal dimension, respectively.

6 Conclusions

In this study, we propose an algorithm to find the differential features by which to tell breast cancer patients from normal people via using the Prim MST algorithm to cluster features of breast cancer data set (WDBC), and selecting the features which are strongly related to the class labels from each cluster to form the differential feature subset. We then propose to find the optimum number of feature clusters by using the F-statistics of a clustering. The similarities between features and the similarities between features and class labels are measured by cosine similarity or Pearson correlation coefficient when finding the differential features. The similarities between samples are measured by cosine similarity, Pearson correlation coefficient or Euclidean distance when group the samples into two clusters via MST clustering algorithm. The clustering accuracy of MST clustering algorithm on WDBC samples with the selected differential features are calculated and compared with that of MST with samples including all of original 30 features and that of available related algorithms.

The experimental results demonstrate that the proposed approach can find the differential features of features 1, 10, and 20 whose meanings are mean radius, mean fractal dimension, and standard error of fractal dimension respectively. The recognized differential features can lead the highest clustering accuracy of MST algorithm on breast cancer dataset when the similarities between features and the similarities between features and class labels are both measured by cosine similarity, and the similarities between samples are measured by Euclidean distance. The clustering accuracy of MST algorithm with the differential features are advanced about 14 % compared to that of samples with all of original 30 features. However, the clustering accuracy of MST algorithm on breast cancer data set with recognized differential features is not as high as those of compared algorithms'.

Therefore the differential feature recognition algorithm based on F-statistics and MST algorithm need further research, and we have done some researches of it by using other clustering algorithm such as those based on densities instead of the MST clustering algorithm. We will show the further research results in other publications.

Acknowledgements. We are much obliged to those who share the datasets in the machine learning repository of UCI. This work is supported in part by the National Natural Science Foundation of China under Grant No. 61673251, is also supported by the Key Science and

Technology Program of Shaanxi Province of China under Grant No. 2013K12-03-24, and is at the same time supported by the Fundamental Research Funds for the Central Universities under Grant No. GK201503067 and 2016CSY009, and by the Innovation Funds of Graduate Programs at Shaanxi Normal University under Grant No. 2015CXS028.

References

1. Jiaqing, Z., Shu, W., Xinming, Q.: The present situation and version of breast cancer. Chin. J. Surg. **40**(3), 161 (2002)
2. Magendiran, N., Jayaranjani, J.: An efficient fast clustering-based feature subset selection algorithm for high-dimensional data. Int. J. Innov. Res. Sci. Eng. Technol. **3**(1), 405–408 (2014)
3. Yan, W., Wu, W.: Data Structure in C, pp. 173–176. Tsinghua University Press, Beijing (2007)
4. Xie, J., Liu, C.: Fuzzy Mathematics Method and its Application, 2nd edn. Huazhong University of Science & Technology Press, Wuhan (2000)
5. Xinbo, G., Jie, L., Dacheng, T., et al.: Fuzziness measurement of fuzzy sets and its application in cluster validity analysis. Int. J. Fuzzy Syst. **9**(4), 188–197 (2007)
6. Huang, Z., Michael, K.Ng.: A fuzzy k-modes algorithm for clustering categorical data. IEEE Trans. Fuzzy Syst. **4**(7), 446–452 (1999)
7. Xie, J., Zhou, Y.: A new criterion for clustering algorithm. J. Shaanxi Norm. Univ. (Nat. Sci. Ed.) **43**(6), 1–8 (2015)
8. Tan, P.N., Steinbach, M., Kumar, V.: An introduction to data mining, pp. 65–83. China Machine Press, Beijing (2010)
9. UCI Machine Learning Repository [DB/OL], 24 March 2016. http://mlr.cs.umass.edu/ml/datasets/Breast+Cancer+Wisconsin+%28Diagnostic%29
10. Li, W., Xianzhong, Z., Jie, S.: An improved rough k-means clustering algorithm. Control Decis. **27**(11), 1711–1719 (2012)
11. Jiyu, L., Qiang, W., Hao, S., Lvyun, Z.: Weighted KNN data classification algorithm based on rough set. Comput. Sci. **42**(10), 281–286 (2015)
12. Fan, M., Li, Z., Shi, X.: A clustering algorithm based on local center object. Comput. Eng. Sci. **36**(9), 1611–1616 (2014)
13. Qing, M., Juanying, X.: New k-medoids clustering algorithm based on granular computing. J. Comput. Appl. **32**(7), 1973–1977 (2012)

Author Index

Printed in the United States
By Bookmasters